More Praise for Dr. Walter
Back to Health by Choice

"Dr. Walter Salubro has a passion to help people live more fully. This book is a must read for everyone. If you want to live healthier and live longer, apply the principles that he teaches."

—Dr. Andrew Scott, DC
Chiropractor
Coauthor, *Abundance With Ease*

"If you allow it, *Back to Health by Choice* has the potential to change and even save your life from a quality of life perspective. I am specifically intrigued and passionate about the emphasis on the importance of choices that we make regarding our health care. I encourage you to take this book and read it from the perspective of taking action steps that you need to take to correct and preserve the life potential that you possess. Your actions today will determine your future health in 20 to 30 years, and you have a possibility and opportunity to change it now based on the knowledge and wisdom that Dr. Walter Salubro offers in this book."

—Dr. Dmitri Sokolov, DC
Chiropractor
Awarded "Worldwide Leader in Health Care" in 2012 by the International Association of Health Care Practitioners

"I remember the first time I met Dr. Walter Salubro. Dr. Walter Salubro is energetic, caring, and very detailed in his approach with anything. The care he takes with his patients is unparalleled, and the stories he reveals in his book are a must read. I would trust Dr. Salubro with my mom, sister, dad, or brother in a heartbeat. His passion and vigor for healing is palpable in this book. Reading *Back to Health by Choice* got me even more excited to help patients and change lives for the next day. This book is a must read for chiropractors and patients alike."

—Dr. Jeremy Weisz, DC
Chiropractor
Founder of Chiropractical Solutions

Back to Health
by Choice

W. Toth   Dec 5/2015.

Back to Health by Choice

How to Relieve Pain, Conquer Stress,
and Supercharge Your Health
the Chiropractic Way

Walter Salubro, DC
Maple, ON

Back to Health by Choice
How to Relieve Pain, Conquer Stress, and Supercharge
Your Health the Chiropractic Way
By Walter Salubro, DC

Ordering Information
Books can be ordered directly from Walter Salubro:
Tel: 905-303-1009   Fax: 905-303-1071
orders@waltersalubro.com
www.WalterSalubro.com

ISBN 978-0-9947913-0-6

First Edition

Library and Archives Canada Cataloguing in Publication

Salubro, Walter, 1973- author
        Back to health by choice : how to relieve pain, conquer stress,
and supercharge your health the chiropractic way / Walter Salubro,
DC.

Includes bibliographical references and index.
Issued in print and audio format.
ISBN 978-0-9947913-0-6 (paperback).--ISBN 978-0-9947913-1-3 (audiobook)

        1. Chiropractic. 2. Pain--Alternative treatment. 3. Stress (Psychology)--
Alternative treatment. I. Title.

RZ241.S24 2015   615.5'34   C2015-903967-3
                                                              C2015-903968-1

This book is dedicated to
the loving memories of
my cousin Dr. Antonio Taverniti
and my friend Dr. Tony Spataro.

Contents

Disclaimer

The information provided in this book is intended for information purposes only and does not constitute medical, chiropractic, health, or other advice of any kind or nature. The information provided is strictly for educational purposes. The reading or receiving of information in this book does not create an advisory relationship of any nature. If you apply information in this book, you take full responsibility for your actions or inactions. This book is not meant to be used, nor should it be used, to address, diagnose, or treat any medical condition of any kind or nature. This book is not intended as a substitute for the medical advice of physicians or the professional advice of any other health-care practitioner. The reader or recipient of information in this book should regularly consult a physician and/or his or her primary health-care provider in matters relating to their health. This book does not contain all information available regarding the subjects addressed in this book. This book has not been created to be specific to any individual's needs. Every effort has been made to make this book as accurate as possible. However, there may be typographical and/or content errors or omissions. This book may contain information that is out-of-date, inaccurate, or inapplicable. The author has, and shall have, no liability or responsibility whatsoever to any person or entity regarding any matter related to this book and/or its contents, including without limiting the generality of the foregoing, any loss or damage incurred, or alleged to have been incurred, directly or indirectly, in relation to the information, or application or nonapplication of the information, contained in this book. If you do not wish to be bound by the disclaimer set out on this page, you may return this book to the author/publisher for a full refund (on proof of purchase).

About the Author

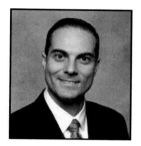 Dr. Walter Salubro is a family wellness chiropractor and the owner of Back To Health Chiropractic Centre in Maple, Ontario. He grew up in Toronto, Ontario, and moved to Vaughan, Ontario, with his family at the age of fifteen.

Dr. Salubro graduated from York University in 1996 and from the National College of Chiropractic in 1999. He has been practicing chiropractic and serving his community of Maple and Vaughan for over fifteen years.

Dr. Salubro provides chiropractic care to people of all age groups. He is trained in applying specific chiropractic techniques that are just as suitable for children as they are for adults. In addition to offering specific spinal adjustments and posture corrective techniques, Dr. Salubro offers an extensive lineup of health seminars, exercise classes, and a run/walk club to his patients. Dr. Salubro is an avid runner, having completed multiple marathons and half marathons.

Dr. Walter Salubro is dedicated to providing exceptional chiropractic care for all his patients. He caters to the care of infants and pregnant mothers. Dr. Salubro is certified from the Academy of Chiropractic Family Practice and the Council on Chiropractic Pediatrics (CACCP). Dr. Walter Salubro is Webster Technique Certified, which is certified and recognized by the International Chiropractic Pediatric Association (ICPA).

Foreword

As a full-time practicing chiropractor, and an international speaker and lecturer, I take tremendous pride in delivering detailed and effective teaching material. I first met Dr. Walter Salubro many years ago when he attended my Thompson Technique Seminars in Toronto. Dr. Salubro was an avid learner and dedicated practitioner striving to be the very best in the seminar so that he could better serve his patients. His drive was tremendous, but it was secondary to his overwhelming kindness and good nature.

Once Dr. Salubro became certified in my seminar series, there was no doubt in my mind that I wanted him as one of my assistant instructors to help teach upcoming students and doctors who attended the program. Walter is one of my finest assistant instructors and always goes above and beyond in every capacity. I am honored to call him a colleague and friend.

With that said, it is my pleasure to introduce this new book: *Back to Health by Choice*. I love the title because health is very much a choice. What we choose to do every day in our lives affects our health in a very significant capacity. Dr. Walter eloquently explains how chiropractic approaches health in a vitalistic way, incorporating both the physical body as well as the innate energy that controls every cell, tissue, and organ. The chiropractic case studies that are presented are moving, educational, and inspirational and reinforce the power of the chiropractic adjustment and chiropractic lifestyle in optimizing health in all patients, regardless of their individual case.

Dr. Salubro goes on to explain, in an easily understood format, the nature of stress, the overwhelming role that it has on our health, and how chiropractic deals with this epidemic problem.

I have great respect for the time, dedication, and effort Dr. Salubro put into the creation of this book. The energy that he expended is evident with each page that is read.

In my opinion, this book will help the general public understand chiropractic better and, most importantly, will help them understand that their health is in their hands. Their health is ultimately their choice.

I am proud of you, Walter. Proud of the work you put into this book, and proud to call you a friend.

Dr. John Minardi, BHK, DC
Chiropractor, speaker, author
The Complete Thompson Textbook:
Minardi Integrated Systems

Acknowledgments

It has always been a dream of mine to author a book. Such an undertaking cannot be accomplished without the inspiration of other people. At this time, I wish to acknowledge the people who have directly and indirectly inspired me and assisted me throughout my life and my chiropractic journey. Part of this journey is the writing of this book.

First and foremost, I thank my mom, Teresa, and my dad, Giuseppe, for believing in me, for trusting me with all my life and career decisions, and for all their love and support.

I am grateful to my siblings, Enea, Sigfrido and Stella, for all their love and support.

I am grateful to my fiancée and soon-to-be wife, Micheline, for her continuous support and encouragement in writing this book.

I am so thankful for my late cousin, Dr. Tony Taverniti, who has always been a guide, inspiration, and mentor for me from day one of my chiropractic journey. Whenever I had a challenge or a question, my cousin, Dr. Taverniti, was always there to guide me in the right direction.

I am grateful to my Aunt Teresa, my cousin Francesca, and my cousin Anna for their support throughout my chiropractic journey.

All of my life lessons and inspirations have resulted from being a chiropractor. And for this reason I am thoroughly grateful for the chiropractic profession as a whole; for my alma mater, National College of Chiropractic (now called National University of Health Sciences); for D. D. Palmer, the founder of chiropractic; for his son, B. J. Palmer the developer of chiropractic; for all the pioneer chiropractors; and for all the chiropractic leaders and teachers of today.

I am grateful for Dr. Joseph Oliva, who gave me my first start in his office as a chiropractic associate in my early days.

I am so grateful for my late friend, Dr. Tony Spataro, who, when I was experiencing a change of direction in my life and in my career in 2004, allowed me to join and practice in his chiropractic office. Dr. Spataro was a great chiropractor and an equally great friend. I learned a lot from him. Dr. Spataro was the first chiropractor to lead me to principled chiropractic care.

There are so many chiropractors who have been an integral part of my learning and growth as a chiropractic doctor. In no particular order, I wish to acknowledge them here as well.

I am grateful for Dr. Joel Weisberg, who has been a valuable chiropractic mentor to me over the years.

I am thankful for Dr. Peter Amlinger for being a leader in teaching about principled chiropractic. I am so grateful I have attended his Pure and Powerful Seminars and for all his amazing chiropractic speakers. It is in his Pure and Powerful Seminars that I have rekindled my chiropractic healing principles.

I am grateful to Dr. Gilles Lamarche for his profound teachings during his lectures and teleconferences. They have made a big impact in leading me to being a principled chiropractor.

I am grateful for Dr. Tom Preston, who was the first to acknowledge my writing skills and that I had it in me to author a book. That meant so much to me. Thank you for all your guidance and coaching.

I am grateful to Dr. Ryan French, Dr. Mark Foullong, Dr. Trevor Middleton, and Dr. Andrew Scott for their coaching and guidance and for inspiring me to be a principled family chiropractor.

I am thankful to my good friend Dr. Jeremy Weisz for his encouragement, motivation, and accountability and for all the inspiring brainstorming conversations we have shared.

I am grateful for Dr. Yurij Chewpa and Dr. Ed Quirk, who, with their Warrior Coaching, have helped me chisel away many blocks to my personal and professional growth and success.

I am grateful for all my chiropractic technique teachers. Special thanks go out to Dr. John Minardi, who trained me in the Thompson Technique. Through his Thompson Technique Seminars, I have become more certain and skilled at assessing for and correcting vertebral subluxations. I am also grateful for Dr. Deed Harrison, who, through his trainings and seminars, has given me an understanding and a solid foundation to the Chiropractic Biophysics® technique and its corrective care protocols.

I am grateful to Dr. Jeanne Ohm and the International Chiropractic Pediatric Association (ICPA), for what the ICPA stands for, and for all its teachers. Through their teachings and seminars, I transformed my chiropractic practice into a family wellness office that cares for people of all ages, including infants, children and pregnant women.

I am thoroughly grateful to my good friend and personal chiropractor, Dr. Dmitri Sokolov, for keeping me subluxations free and healthy with weekly adjustments. Thank you for your guidance and inspiration and for all the thoughtful and enjoyable conversations we have.

I am grateful to all my chiropractic health assistants past and present who have served by my side. You are an integral part of our patients' care and healing journey. Thank you for serving our chiropractic mission and vision.

And last, but certainly not least, I am so grateful for all my patients—past, present, and future. You are the reason why my chiropractic mission is alive today. You are the reason why I am a chiropractor. You have shown me what healing is. You have inspired me to help greater numbers of people. You have inspired me to write this book. I thank you for your trust and for the trust you have given me with your children, your babies, and other members of your family. You, my patients, have led me to continue my chiropractic education in science and philosophy, to sharpen my chiropractic adjusting techniques, and to be principled with my chiropractic care so that I may serve and help more and more people like yourself. As your life has transformed under my chiropractic care, so has mine. Thank you, and I wish you continued health and blessings.

Introduction

Ever since I was a young boy, I always had this innate drive to help people. I recall when other kids got hurt on the playground during school recess, I would immediately go to their assistance. I would do the same when my younger siblings got hurt while playing. I wouldn't know until later in life that I was called to be in a healing profession.

I remember vividly the first time I was introduced to chiropractic. I was thirteen years old. My father was already seeing a chiropractor for back pain. He was off from work at that time so my sister, my brother, and I would tag along with him when he went to his chiropractic appointments.

One day, during my dad's visit to the chiropractor, after his adjustment, he spontaneously asked the chiropractor, "What about my children? Can they get checked and adjusted?"

The chiropractor replied yes. And with that, at the age of thirteen, I received my first chiropractic checkup and adjustment.

Whenever my dad went for his chiropractic adjustments, so did I and my younger siblings. The visit to the chiropractor soon became a familiar occurrence in my life, even though for me it started with wellness chiropractic care.

However, when I was fourteen years old, in grade nine, I started getting severe headaches to the point where I could not focus, concentrate, or do any school work. Instead of taking drugs or going to our family medical doctor for my headaches, I did the only thing I was familiar with—go see my chiropractor. Somehow, even at a young age, I innately knew chiropractic was what I needed for my headaches.

Whenever I had a headache episode, I would simply tell my mom and dad that I was going to see the chiropractor the next day after school. And so, after school, at the age of fourteen, I would take a five-kilometer public bus ride through the city of Toronto to my chiropractor's office, receive my chiropractic adjustment, and then take a seven-kilometer bus ride from the chiropractic office to my home. And I would do that as often as I needed it. I used to love going to my chiropractic appointments. It was an integral part of my life and my well-being from an early age.

I recall when I was eighteen years old, in grade twelve, and it was time to start thinking about university and my future career. I was thinking of becoming an accountant, but I was not really inspired by it. My physics teacher wanted me to become an engineer. That too did not inspire me. So one day, I was sitting on the sofa with my cousin, Dr. Tony Taverniti, who at that time was a recent chiropractic graduate, and he asked me, "Walter, what are you going to do for a career?"

I replied, "Well, I was thinking about accounting."

He noticed that in giving my answer, I wasn't completely aligned with becoming an accountant.

That's when he said, "Why don't you consider being a chiropractor?"

And in that instant, my face immediately lit up. I sat upright and proudly said, "Yes, that's what I'll do, I'll become a chiropractor!"

Even though I had experience with chiropractic as a patient, I don't know why it wasn't even on my radar screen as a profession. But with that suggestion by my cousin, Tony, I was immediately inspired by the idea of becoming a chiropractor.

From that point on, my primary aim in life as I was going through university was to become a chiropractor. In December of 1999, I accomplished my vision and dream when I graduated from the National College of Chiropractic in Lombard, Illinois (a suburb of Chicago).

I truly believe I was called to be a chiropractor. Sometimes in life, you need a little nudge to guide you to your calling. For me, that nudge came from my cousin Tony.

Over my years as a chiropractor, my purpose and conviction in this healing art have grown stronger and stronger. The more I saw healing and transformation in my patients, the more I knew I was fulfilling my calling and purpose as a chiropractor.

I have seen many patients start, continue and succeed with chiropractic care. Their pain was alleviated, their health improved, and they created a transformation in their quality of life.

However, strangely enough, I have also noticed that there were some patients who didn't start their chiropractic care and therefore could not achieve the same level of success with their health as those patients who did.

This led me to ask this question, "Why do some patients start chiropractic and get well while some patients do not start chiropractic care and remain sick?"

What I discovered over much reflection on this question is that the difference comes down to one key factor, and that is *choice*.

Patients who choose healing start their care and get healthier. Patients who do not choose healing do not start their care and stay sick.

That's when I realized that those people who regained their health did so by choice. They got back to health by choice.

And so I made it my mission to help sick and suffering people get well with chiropractic care by leading them to make a choice for healing so they could ultimately live a long-lasting, healthy, happy, and active life.

As you read this book, you will learn about Mary and will follow her healing journey. As you read, keep in mind that "Mary" could very well be you or someone you know, like your mom, dad, brother, sister, aunt, uncle, cousin, friend, neighbor, or coworker.

There are so many "Marys" in this world who are seeking guidance and looking for healing. But there must be a choice first, a choice for healing. Then the form of healing that is congruent with that choice will show up. And for many people, chiropractic is one form of healing they can accept based on their personal values, beliefs, and paradigms.

Also, as you read this book, keep this question in your conscious mind: "How can my life and my health change when I make a choice for healing?" Write this question down on a blank sheet of paper. When the answers come to you, write them down as well.

This one question alone, when earnestly asked and answered, can lead you to a remarkable journey of long-lasting health and happiness.

To your long-lasting health!

Dr. Walter Salubro, DC

www.iBTHCC.com

Free book updates, educational videos, and patient resources

This book is *interactive.*

To read more patient stories, get free chiropractic patient resources, view educational videos, and get access to updates to this book when new versions or editions are released,

visit:

www.BackToHealthByChoice.com/BookBonus

It is the mindful lifestyle
choices you make today
that will keep you healthy,
strong, and enduring
for the marathon called life.

—Walter Salubro

1

Chiropractic and Pain Relief

It was a sunny Monday, and I had just finished with my morning patient visits when Mary quietly and slowly trudged through my clinic's front door. There was something noticeable about Mary when I first set my eyes on her. Trailing right behind Mary was her husband.

It was very evident upon seeing Mary that she was in distress. She had weary eyes, she looked exhausted and her posture was drooping. There was something else about her. She looked like a woman who was on her last straw in life.

In a faint voice, she said, "I've been getting headaches. Can chiropractic help?"

I replied, "Yes! Many people with headaches have benefited from chiropractic care. Before I know if chiropractic is right for you, we need to start with a consultation and examination so we can determine what's causing your headaches."

With that, I immediately noticed a shift in Mary's demeanor. But I'll return to Mary's story in a moment.

Thousands of "Marys" walk into chiropractic offices around the world every day of the week, and what do you think is the most common reason that brings people to a chiropractic office? It's pain.

> ⌘
>
> **Chiropractic has offered millions of people a natural approach for pain relief.**

Many people go to a chiropractor for pain relief. It may be relief from back pain, neck pain, headaches, or some type of joint pain.

People choose chiropractic for pain relief because it works. Chiropractic has offered millions of people a natural approach for pain relief.

Pain can be debilitating. Oftentimes pain can slow you down and affect your quality of life. Someone with back pain, for instance, may have trouble standing for long periods of time. Someone with neck pain may have difficulty sitting and reading. Someone with headaches may have challenges with focus and concentration.

Think about that for a moment. These are simple, everyday activities that are affected by painful conditions. Sometimes you take these daily activities for granted until one day you are stopped in your tracks with a pounding headache or a sore back.

Many people are frustrated with their pain. Many people have suffered for years—and for many of those years they have felt quite alone in believing that no one really understood what they were going through. I see this every week with the people who walk into my office.

Just this week, a woman came to me for help with her back pain. She told me she had been suffering from back pain for seventeen years. Seventeen years of back pain!

She had been to many doctors, was given pain medications, and even tried other forms of therapy. But she still had low-back pain. When I showed her the X-rays of her spine, she started crying. Her spinal X-rays showed severe, advanced degeneration.

She was crying because she had been searching for answers and a solution to her back pain for seventeen years. By the time she came to me, she had a degenerated spine, little strength in her legs, and difficulty walking. No one gave her the solution and the answers she needed. More importantly, no one gave her the solution to correct her back problem.

This has been an all-too-familiar scenario I have encountered with many patients. People search for answers, and oftentimes after many visits to many different specialists and doctors, they never receive the answers that are right for them.

Many people literally search for and try everything under the sun and yet are still stuck with their pain condition or health problem. So they settle for thinking there is no hope for improvement or healing.

The sad and unfortunate part of this is that many people end up saying something such as, "I will probably have this back pain for the rest of my life," "I guess I have to learn to live with it," or "I was told my headache is normal."

> ⌘
>
> **Behind every pain condition there is a subconscious search for healing.**

No! Headaches are not normal.

No! You don't have to have back pain for the rest of your life.

And *no!* You don't have to settle and learn to live with your pain.

This is not a way to go through life. Do you agree? What happens is you continue to suffer—physically, mentally, and emotionally.

The impact is huge, and it translates to a low quality of life stacked with a heap of progressive, chronic health problems. However, it doesn't have to be this way.

From my experience in caring for patients for over fifteen years, I have seen that behind every pain condition is a true lack in quality of life. And yet, behind every pain condition, there is a subconscious search for healing.

I have noticed that pain is what motivates people to take initial action in search of relief, but what they are really searching for, at a subconscious level, is healing.

I had a sense Mary was in search of something more than pain relief, even though pain was what brought her into my office that sunny morning. In the consultation room, I had an opportunity to get to know Mary.

Mary was forty-two years old and a mother of two children—twelve years and eight years of age. Both she and her husband were hard workers doing the best they could to support their children.

Mary told me that fifteen years earlier she had started a new job as an account manager that involved sitting and working at the phone and computer all day. She said that a few months after starting her new job, she began to get headaches.

Mary suffered with headaches for fifteen years. She told me that life had been quite stressful and overwhelming over the years, which aggravated the headaches she was experiencing.

I noticed that Mary squinted her eyes a lot while she was talking to me and that she could barely project her voice beyond a whisper. It was evident to me that she was suffering and in a lot of pain. Many times her husband had to cut in and continue her sentence as she rubbed her forehead to cope with her headache.

Mary went on to tell me that her headaches had been getting worse and worse over the years. She had been to her family doctor and was given pain medications. Even though the painkillers offered her some relief, she said that whenever she stopped taking the medications, her headaches would come back.

As she continued, Mary described her headache as a continuous pounding feeling. She said that in the past several weeks, her headaches had been so severe that she brought herself to the emergency room.

I remember thinking to myself, as I had seen many people with headaches in my office, *What could the hospital possibly do for a woman with headaches?*

The hospital is typically a place that takes care of people in emergencies or crises. The hospital is not meant to be an outpatient clinic, like a doctor's office where someone would typically go for a headache.

Well, Mary told me that she was checked in and then the hospital doctor ran a battery of tests on her. Then she said that they kept her there for three days.

That's when I thought to myself, *Mary has a husband, has a family with two children, has to work a demanding job...where is her quality of life when she's spending three days in the hospital because of her headaches? More importantly, where will her quality of life be in twenty years if she continues on this course?"*

I was curious to hear about her hospital test results, and Mary said, "All my test results came back normal."

I then asked Mary, "Well, did the doctor tell you what's causing your headaches?"

She replied, "No. The doctor did not."

That's when I asked her, "But what did they do in the hospital to help you with your headaches?"

She said, "They sent me home, but before I left the hospital room, they gave me a morphine pill for my headache."

In my thoughts I was shouting, *Morphine pill? Really?*

So I completed Mary's chiropractic examination, which involved assessing her posture and her range of motion and checking for shifts in her spine (called vertebral subluxations) that could be stressing her nervous system. I recommended we take X-rays so we could get a better picture of any damage to her spine. I told Mary I would have to analyze her exam and X-ray findings before I could tell her if chiropractic could help. So she scheduled for her report of findings visit.

Mary had been suffering from headaches for fifteen years! How about you? What has been the main health challenge in your life?

Do you have back pain? Do you have neck pain? Do you suffer from headaches?

Or have you been suffering from other ailments or conditions, like arm pain, leg pain, or numbness and tingling?

Whatever your health challenge, how long have you had it for? One year? Three years? Five years? More than five years? Is that OK with you?

Where will your quality of life or your quality of health be in twenty years if you continue on the same path you are on now?

These are important questions to ask yourself as you continue to read this book.

Many people think it's "normal" to have back pain or neck pain or headaches because they have had the pain for such a long time.

Do you think it's normal?

The reality is that many people don't know what feeling great or normal is anymore because they are so used to living with their pain.

They live with the pain until, one day, they have reached their threshold and, like Mary, can no longer resist the pain and the suffering.

As Mary was leaving the consultation room, I could tell she was a woman in search of something. Pain brought her into my chiropractic office, and she certainly wanted relief from her fifteen years of pounding headaches, but she was in search of something more. She didn't use any of these words, but it was quite clear to me that Mary was in search of *hope*, in search of *reassurance,* and in search of *healing.*

The question for me was, "Is Mary ready to make that choice for healing?" I wouldn't know until after her report of findings visit.

2

A Choice for Healing

I have seen this pattern over and over again in patients. Pain motivates people to seek relief. They are subconsciously seeking healing. And then they are faced with a choice. It's a choice for healing: To choose or not to choose? That is the question. I have found that the answer to that question always comes from within.

Several years ago, I introduced a new patient orientation class during my report of findings visit. Since the introduction of this class, I started to notice something very odd. I noticed that I could have two patients sitting next to each other in my new patient class; one patient starts chiropractic care and will get healthier, and what do you think happens to the other patient? Not much. In fact, the person gets sicker.

This point always reminds me of John. John was a forty-eight year old man who came to my office with back pain. Not only did John have back pain, but he weighed over 300 pounds; had short, shallow breathing; was sweating profusely; had a history of diabetes and a heart condition; and he was taking six different medications every day. John was a sick man.

John came in and instantly said, "All I want is to get rid of my back pain."

Remember, pain is usually the motivating, driving force that finally gets people to take action in search of relief. But whatever John was doing in his life, whatever choices he was making, got him to that point in time with all his current health problems.

I recall saying to myself, *I'm glad John is here in my office because now we can lead him to better health the chiropractic way.*

Well, like with Mary and all my new patients, we always start with a consultation and examination and then proceed to the report of findings visit. The report of findings visit, which in our office includes a new patient orientation class, is always the most important and most transformational visit.

After the class session, the patients get their individual results and recommendations, and if they choose, they start their care. It is my objective to always give our patients all the information they need to make an empowered and informed choice for their own healing and health care.

Well, John too was given this opportunity; however, he kept saying that all he wanted was pain relief. His examination and X-ray findings all pointed to the fact that the pain was not the problem.

Instead, he had an underlying spinal condition, called vertebral subluxation (also referred to as spinal misalignment), that was causing the pain. The vertebral subluxations had to be addressed and corrected for proper healing to be optimized.

With that correction, of course, comes the relief of pain. But the pain relief comes as a result of correcting the underlying spinal condition (the vertebral subluxations) with specific, scientific chiropractic adjustments.

> ⌘
>
> **Until you make a choice for healing, nothing happens.**

John received his first chiropractic adjustment but didn't follow through with the rest of the recommendations. He never returned to continue his care. It was clear that his choice for healing did not extend past his search for instant pain relief. To my sadness, I found out a year later that John suffered a massive heart attack and passed away.

You see, you can have access to the greatest health care in the world, but until you make a choice for healing, nothing happens. Healing always starts from within, and it starts when you make that choice, a choice for healing.

And so, in my chiropractic office, we lead and guide patients to make a choice for healing, and when they make that choice, we start noticing people become healthier, happier, and they begin experiencing a higher quality of life.

It's hard to imagine why someone would not commit to his or her own health and well-being. But I can say that it does happen.

There is always that moment of truth when someone is faced with making a decision and must ask this question: "Am I ready to commit to my health or not?"

You see, commitments are not easy. A commitment to health and wellness requires a complete shift in everything you have been doing in your life. It requires a shift in your eating habits. It requires a shift in your physical activity. It requires a shift in addressing and managing your stress. It requires a shift in setting life goals and creating an ideal life vision.

As you learn more about chiropractic, you will see that it also requires a shift in choosing the chiropractic way to better health. The chiropractic way to better health is keeping your spine optimized and your nervous system healthy.

Through the years of caring for many people at my office with chiropractic care, I have seen three distinct scenarios when it comes to a choice for healing:

1. Some people choose healing without hesitation. This means that they are ready, and consequently that their life and their health will be transformed.

2. Some people need more guidance and direction before choosing healing. They are borderline ready. It just means there are blocks in the way that need to be removed; and with the proper guidance, they'll

choose healing. They too will experience a transformation in their life and their health.

3. Some people are just not ready to choose healing. For instance, some people may be attached to their pain condition, they may fear change, or they may fear losing their identity as a sick and suffering person. Or they may have other blocks that interfere with their choice for healing. However, without a choice for healing, nothing will change for them. They will continue on their current path in life—a path of pain, illness, and suffering. Unfortunately, some people may never make a choice for healing.

I have come to realize that, at a subconscious level, people have already decided which direction they will take even before I meet them. But I will never know until I guide them through our initial visit and then our report of findings visit.

> ⌘
>
> **A doctor can only lead, direct, educate, and give best opinions and recommendations but in the end, patients must make the choice for their health and their healing.**

I can't make that choice for patients. No doctor can. A doctor can only lead, direct, educate, and give their best opinions and recommendations, but in the end, the patients must make the choice for their health and their healing.

For instance, if a doctor tells a patient to quit smoking because smoking could cause cancer and heart disease, whose choice is it to quit smoking? That's right! It's the patient's choice. The same is true for all other health-related choices.

I have also realized that many other health-care modalities can represent a choice for healing for people, but since I am a chiropractor, I can only truly talk about my chiropractic experience with patients. And so, for many people, chiropractic represents a choice for the specific form of healing that is congruent with their personal values, beliefs, and paradigms.

With regards to Mary, I wasn't quite sure which way she would choose until her report of findings visit. But I was eager to give her the results and recommendations because, after having analyzed her X-rays and identified her vertebral subluxations, I saw that indeed she was a good candidate for chiropractic care and that chiropractic could help her.

Mary showed up to my new patient orientation class with her husband by her side for support. I have noticed, too, that when a patient has the support of a spouse or a family member, this support considerably favors and assists with their healing and recovery. Because we want to create the best opportunity for our patients' healing and recovery, we encourage our patients to bring their spouses to their report of findings visit.

Mary listened attentively during the orientation class. When the class session was over, my assistant brought Mary and her husband to the private consultation room for a report of her X-ray findings. Even before I could say hello, Mary politely interrupted me and started speaking in her now familiar soft voice:

"Dr. Walter, I had to go back to the emergency room because my headache was so severe that I didn't know what else to do."

I replied, "What did they do for you at the hospital this time?"

She said, "They gave me a morphine injection and then sent me home."

Again in my thoughts, but with more fury this time, I was screaming, *A morphine injection? Is this the best our health-care system can do for this woman who is losing quality of life because of headaches?*

I remained calm and said, "I see. Well, I'm glad we took your X-rays because I did find a problem in your spinal alignment, but the good news is we can help."

I proceeded to show her the neck X-rays, which confirmed a major shifting in the normal alignment of her spine as well as damage in the form of degenerative arthritis.

Over time, when spinal misalignments (vertebral subluxations) persist and are not detected and corrected, they will proceed to cause damage and degeneration to the bones and discs of the spine.

I explained to Mary how the misalignment in her neck created tension on her spinal cord and nerves and how it was causing her headaches because the nerves of the neck travel to the area of the head.

I reassured Mary that we could help make corrections but that it would take some time, some effort, and a commitment on her part.

Mary was relieved because, for the first time in fifteen years, someone finally told her what the problem was, what was causing her headaches, that there was an opportunity for correcting the underlying problem, and that there was hope for healing.

> ⌘
>
> **When spinal misalignments (vertebral subluxations) persist, they cause damage and degeneration to the bones and discs of the spine.**

But I still wasn't sure what her decision would be for starting chiropractic care and for following through with the recommendations. I didn't know yet if she had made a choice for healing.

I proceeded, "Mary, this will take a commitment on your part. Is chiropractic care something you want to commit to? Is your health important enough to commit to getting your spine corrected?"

This may sound like a strange question to ask, but really, every patient is different, and I don't know the extent of someone's commitment to getting healthy until I ask. But it is at this moment of asking, this moment of truth, that I truly discover the person's choice for healing.

The patient's answer always comes from within. Deep down inside, every patient knows the answer. But is the patient ready for it? Is the patient ready for healing?

To my delight, Mary was ready, and she did make a choice for healing. How did I know?

I knew because, in that moment, she answered, "Yes, I am ready to commit to my health."

You see, making that initial choice is crucial and necessary to get the process started because it gets you on that path for healing. And commitment is what keeps you on that path.

Nothing gets started in life without an initial choice. But starting is not enough; to see results, you must follow through, and a solid commitment is essential for follow through.

I was excited for Mary, as with all my patients who choose chiropractic care, because I knew it would create a transformation in her life. She might not have known it at that time, but I have seen it over and over again with all my other patients who have chosen chiropractic as their form for healing.

I have seen lives transformed with chiropractic. I have seen people laugh more in life with chiropractic. I have seen people adapt to stresses better with chiropractic. I have seen people's health improve with chiropractic.

I have seen people's energy elevate with chiropractic. I have seen people's mood go from depression to joy for life with chiropractic.

I have seen people start to enjoy a better quality of life with chiropractic. I have seen people create a loving family bond with chiropractic. But it all starts with a choice—a choice for healing.

3

More than Pain Relief

How someone defines his or her quality of life is unique for each and every person. People tend to go to a chiropractor because of a specific pain complaint. They continue on with chiropractic care because of the superior quality of life they begin to experience and enjoy. They continue to enjoy a higher quality of life because they made a choice for healing and a choice for their own health and wellness.

Chiropractic care helps get people beyond the pain relief. Chiropractic helps get people beyond the suffering. Chiropractic helps bring back a quality of life in people. When asked about the most significant change our patients have received from chiropractic care, the response given is mostly in relation to improved quality of life and hardly ever about the original pain condition they first came in with.

I had a man come in once with severe neck pain and limited mobility. After eight weeks of chiropractic care we did his progress exam. I asked what his most significant improvement had been since he had started chiropractic care.

Even though he had no more neck pain and had improved mobility, he said that his most significant improvement was that he no longer had heartburn. He went on to say that he could now enjoy eating many more foods he had previously given up because of heartburn and indigestion.

> ⌘
>
> **Chiropractic brings you back to feeling fully alive again. It leads you to your optimal quality of life.**

I recall a woman who came in with back pain. Within weeks of starting chiropractic care, her back pain was improving. However, to her delight, she told me she now had more clarity, had more energy, was feeling more rested, and was inspired to start writing again. Her creativity was sparked, and her passion for writing, which was dormant for years, was ignited again.

There was yet another woman who came in with neck pain, back pain, and shoulder pain. After her first chiropractic visit, she said she had the best sleep of the past five years.

Yes, chiropractic can help with relief of pain. But it offers much more than that. It brings you back to feeling fully alive again. It leads you to your optimal quality of life.

Quality of life may mean something different to each and every individual. For some people quality of life means being able to return to their hockey game because their back is much stronger.

For others, quality of life means being able to return to work so they can continue to support their family.

For a mom, quality of life means being able to feed her one-year-old child with comfort and ease because she can finally lift her arm again.

For a dad, quality of life means finally getting a good night's sleep and waking up feeling refreshed.

For a first-time mother-to-be, quality of life means going through her first pregnancy free of stress, free of back pain, and feeling totally confident, ready and empowered for the birth of her baby.

These represent only a small sample of some of the improvements in quality of life that chiropractic patients have reported.

Chiropractic has been helping people improve their health and quality of life since its discovery by D. D. Palmer in 1895. Consider that the very first chiropractic adjustment was delivered by its founder, D. D. Palmer, with the intention of restoring hearing loss in his patient, Harvey Lillard. And it did! That first chiropractic adjustment did restore Mr. Lillard's hearing.

Chiropractic was founded on vitalistic principles of health and healing, with the intention of supporting the body's natural functions and healing abilities.

D. D. Palmer and other pioneer chiropractors set out to help the sick and the suffering with chiropractic care. They didn't just operate clinics; the early chiropractors operated in infirmaries. They were literary taking care of ill people with chiropractic.

Chiropractic has come a long way since its early pioneer days. I always find it unsettling that chiropractic today is primarily viewed by the public as a pain-relief therapy. Chiropractic offers far more than just pain relief.

When diving into the history of chiropractic, it is evident that chiropractic was not originally founded on, nor was it originally promoted as, a pain-relief therapy.

Some early 1900s chiropractic advertisements depict this clearly. For example, a circa 1921 chiropractic ad had this as one of its headlines: "Chiropractic Adjustments Remove the Cause of So Called"[1]

Underneath this headline the ad listed a myriad of the "so-called" diseases the headline was referring to, which were:

Rheumatism
Asthma
Lumbago
Stomach
Spleen
Liver
Eye Troubles
High Blood Pressure
Nervous and Skin Disorders
Constipation
Headaches

Catarrh
Paralysis
Bronchitis
Neuritis
Deafness
Hay Fever

Another advertisement by an Indianapolis chiropractor in 1930 had this as its headline: "Chiropractic Treatment Reaches the Basic Cause"[2]

The rest of the ad went on to say:

Myriads of disorders are due to mal-adjustments of the vertebrae, the great trunk line of the nervous system. The success of chiropractic treatment in MILLIONS OF CASES is due to its ability to counteract illness at the source. Let it restore YOUR system to its natural healthy vigor.

That's exactly what people are looking for, to live a natural, healthy, quality of life full of vigor.

What a wonderful word, *vigor*. Let's examine the definition of the word *vigor*. According to the *Oxford Dictionary*, the definition of vigor is "physical strength and good health."[3]

The origin of the word vigor comes from the Latin word *vigere*, meaning "be lively."

Wouldn't you want physical strength, good health, and to be lively? That is a great question to ask yourself.

You see, the early chiropractors had it right when they said, "Let chiropractic restore your system to its natural healthy vigor" because chiropractic offers far more than just pain relief.

Yes, pain too will hinder your quality of life. And if pain is what it takes to get introduced to chiropractic care, that is understandable. Know, however, that chiropractic care offers far more than merely pain relief. It helps restore your vigor and ensure your quality of life.

> ⌘
>
> **Chiropractic offers far more than merely pain relief. It helps restore your vigor and ensure your quality of life.**

When quality of life is hindered, you cannot experience bliss, joy, and happiness. Today, as a century ago, regardless of what motivates someone to seek chiropractic, I contend that the person is in search of a transformation in his or her quality of life.

This motive can be at a conscious level or at a subconscious level. Either way, there must first be a choice for healing. Without that choice, nothing can begin to change. The same old pain conditions and health problems will continue to repeat themselves, leading to more stress, more frustration, and more illness unless there is a choice for healing.

After the choice for healing, the next important component necessary in promoting a positive change in quality of life is commitment. A choice is weak without a commitment to back it up.

It's like running in a road race. You can choose to start the run, but without a commitment to cross the finish line, you will never complete the race. It's your commitment that will get you to follow through and to cross the finish line so you can get the result you choose to have.

You can choose healing, you can choose to start chiropractic care, and you can choose to have a higher quality of life. Your choosing will start the process. However, without a commitment to follow through, you can never see results come to fruition. Sticking to your commitment is crucial to your success in life, especially when it comes to your health and well-being.

Mary was finally ready to break her fifteen-year pattern of headaches because she made a conscious choice for healing and a commitment to her care.

The next question that I asked myself was, *Is Mary willing to follow through?*

I have seen many people not receive the full benefits of chiropractic care because they quit too early. They didn't cross the finish line. Was this going to happen to Mary?

It's important to keep in mind this important principle—healing takes time. Many people's health problems and degenerative conditions did not develop in one day. They developed over many years and for some people over decades.

Even if the pain just began a few days earlier, the underlying problem could have been developing for years and years. This is why it's important to think beyond pain-relief care and think in terms of correcting the underlying problem causing the pain. It is the aim of chiropractic to correct the underlying problem causing the pain.

For those people who do follow through with their chiropractic care, they will enjoy many health benefits beyond pain relief. They will enjoy natural, healthy vigor, as you will soon discover.

4

Chiropractic: A Vitalistic Approach to Health

Many years ago when I was attending chiropractic college, one of my teachers, who was also a chiropractor, said this to our study group: "My children have been adjusted since the first day they were born, and so far, they have never had a cold or the flu. Their cousins, who have never received chiropractic care, have all had multiple colds and flus."

To this day, I still can hear my teacher's voice telling this story. Although I have been under chiropractic care since my early years, I really didn't grasp the fundamental essence of chiropractic until many years later when I started seeing the remarkable health changes that had occurred with my own patients.

There are four fundamental principles and self-evident truths upon which chiropractic was founded on. They are...

Fundamental Principle #1

The body has an inborn, innate ability to self-heal and self-regulate.

Fundamental Principle #2

The nervous system is the one system that coordinates and controls the function of all cells, tissues, and organ systems. Said another way, the nervous system controls all bodily functions, all healing, and all repair.

Fundamental Principle #3

Vertebral subluxations (spinal misalignments) are the number one cause of strain and stress on your nervous system, causing interference to your innate ability to function, heal, and repair optimally.

Fundamental Principle #4

Chiropractic is the only health-care profession that is dedicated to locating subluxations with specific spinal analyses and the only profession that is dedicated to correcting subluxations through the chiropractic adjustment. Correcting subluxations removes the interference on the nervous system thereby removing interference on the body's innate ability to function, heal, and repair optimally.

Let's look at the first fundamental principle, which says that the body has an inborn, innate ability to self-heal and self-regulate.

#1

The Body Has an Inborn, Innate Ability to Self-Heal and Self-Regulate

Isn't it intriguing that when you cut or scrape your hand, within seconds, immune cells are fighting off invading bacteria and protecting you from infection, that within hours the wound begins to close and scars over, and that within days it is completely healed?

Isn't it amazing that your body is always maintained at a constant temperature, whether it's hot or cold out? Your body knows how to regulate itself automatically.

The same is true for all your vital organs and systems. Your digestive system intelligently knows how to break down the food you eat, absorb all the necessary vitamins, minerals and nutrients, and get rid of all the waste by-products.

Your lungs are constantly working to get oxygen into your system and expel carbon dioxide.

Your immune system is always ready, on alert, to fight off invading organisms like bacteria and viruses.

Sometimes we take these bodily processes for granted because they occur automatically.

But how does this happen automatically? This happens because your body has an innate ability to self-heal and self-regulate. Your body has an innate ability to remain in balance—in homeostasis. And when this balance is off, your body has an innate ability to restore itself to balance again. All this is possible because your body has a built-in, innate intelligence.

B. J. Palmer, who is the son of D. D. Palmer and is renowned as the developer of the chiropractic profession, says this about innate intelligence in his book, *The Bigness of the Fellow Within:*

> Innate Intelligence (nature, spirit, subconscious or unconscious mind, or other name given to this internal power within us) is what cures and heals. Innate Intelligence is never sick, never depleted, never runs dry. It is an exhaustless reservoir of Intelligence and power and is always full to capacity and running over. It is there, ready, willing, anxious to deliver life and health at all times, in all places, and in all ways. Its potentials are there from the moment of birth to the last breath before death. No matter how sick, run down, depleted, or dying *the body*, the Innate power house is desiring to, capable of, and ready to get the sick body well.[1]

Innate intelligence is present everywhere in your body and directs all matter of the body. In other words, there is an intelligent wisdom within your body that gives life to your body.

It is that innate intelligence that powers and runs your body, and it is that innate intelligence that allows your body to heal. Let's begin to acknowledge the innate intelligence inherent within us.

Now, let's examine the second fundamental principle which says that the nervous system controls all bodily functions, all healing, and all repairs in your body.

#2

The Nervous System Controls All Bodily Functions, All Healing, and All Repairs in Your Body

Both principle one and principle two are closely related. Chiropractic recognizes that innate intelligence is expressed in your body through the nervous system.

Stated another way, chiropractic acknowledges that innate intelligence communicates with all your body parts through all your nerve channels, from brain to spinal cord to spinal nerves to all organs and body parts. The nervous system acts like a communication network that connects all your cells, organs, and tissues so they keep functioning at 100 percent capacity—that is, so they self-heal and self-regulate.

Your built-in innate intelligence gives you survival mechanisms; it is responsible for growth, replication, and reproduction; and it even guides your intuition. When this communication is broken or interfered with, your health and your life is not expressed at its full potential. Think about that for a moment. Do you want to express full health and life potential, or do you want to express less health and life potential?

To have a high quality of life, you need your health to be expressed at its maximum potential, which means you need 100 percent expression of innate intelligence. That's when you are living life to the fullest.

The spinal cord is the main pipeline that feeds life to your entire body; it is the primary connection between brain and body. The spinal cord is well protected by the spinal column. In fact, the primary purpose of the spinal column is to protect the spinal cord, just like the skull protects the brain.

Any damage to the brain can be detrimental and can cause debilitating loss of bodily functions. The same is true for the spinal cord. Any damage to the spinal cord also can be detrimental and can cause debilitating loss of bodily functions. Since the spine protects the spinal cord, it is essential that it is positioned in its optimal alignment so your body can express 100 percent function, 100 percent healing, and 100 percent repair.

The optimal alignment of the spine is straight when viewed from the front (or back), and it has three natural curves when viewed from the side. This is the normal alignment of the spine that chiropractors look for when examining spinal X-rays.

You learned so far that the body is self-healing and self-regulating and that this innate ability to self-heal and self-regulate is communicated by the brain and spinal cord (which make up your central nervous system). The spinal column protects the spinal cord. The spinal cord is the lifeline between your brain (the central "computer") and the rest of your body (your cells, tissues, and organs).

For optimal function and optimal health, the communication from the brain through the spinal cord to all your organs and body parts must be flowing at 100 percent without interference. What causes interference on this nerve flow? Spinal misalignments—also called vertebral subluxations.

This brings us to the third fundamental principle, which says that vertebral subluxations (spinal misalignments) are the number one cause of strain and stress on your nervous system and interfere with your innate ability to function, heal, and repair optimally.

#3

Vertebral Subluxations Place Stress on Your Nervous System and Interfere with Your Innate Ability to Function, Heal, and Repair Optimally

Vertebral subluxations are caused by stress. The source of stress can be physical, chemical, or emotional. Said another way, as D. D. Palmer referred to it, the source of stress can be from trauma, toxins, or thoughts.

> ⌘
>
> An optimal spine means optimal health.

Physical trauma can be either of a minor type, like repetitive strains over time (e.g. sitting in front of a computer at work) or of a major type, like a car accident or a fall. Chemical stress can be from toxins in foods, water, and air. Emotional stress can be from negative thought patterns and relationship problems.

These are only some examples of each source of stress. Regardless of the source of stress—physical, chemical, or emotional—the nervous system will always be affected causing interference in the communication between the brain and the rest of the body.

Therefore, the spine, which protects the spinal cord, must be kept optimized in its natural position. An optimal spine means optimal health.

Getting checked for vertebral subluxations is therefore essential. The only way to determine if you have subluxations is to get a spinal checkup by a chiropractor.

This brings us to the fourth fundamental principle, which says that chiropractic is the only health-care profession that is dedicated to locating vertebral subluxations and correcting subluxations through the chiropractic adjustment, thereby restoring the body's ability to function, heal, and repair optimally.

#4

Chiropractors are Trained for and Dedicated to Locating Vertebral Subluxations and Skilled at Correcting Subluxations through the Chiropractic Adjustment

Vertebral subluxations can cause pain, but oftentimes they do not. So if you have no pain or no symptoms, it doesn't necessarily mean you don't have subluxations that could be interfering with your nervous system.

A chiropractic checkup can help detect subluxations. Once subluxations are located, a chiropractor can help correct them, thereby restoring the spine and nervous system to optimal alignment and optimal function. This leads to a better ability to handle stress, improved sleeping, improved mobility, relief from muscle tension, a quicker return to your daily activities, and an overall improvement in your quality of health and quality of life.

These are some of the amazing benefits chiropractic patients have reported since starting their chiropractic care—because an optimal spine leads to optimal health. Chiropractic is an essential component of health-care for people of all ages, from infants to seniors.

In Mary's case, headaches originally brought her to my chiropractic office. Remember, most people seek help when they are in pain. Pain is a powerful motivator.

In two months, while under chiropractic care, the intensity of Mary's headaches dropped from a 10 to a 3, where 10 is the worst pain on a scale of 0 to 10. By the end of Mary's third month of chiropractic care, she reported that she had no more headaches. In addition, she had stopped taking her pain medications. When we did her annual progress exam, she still reported no more headaches.

Does chiropractic help with pain relief? Yes. Many people experience pain relief with chiropractic care. Chiropractic care for pain relief is natural and safe.

Many people take too many medications for pain relief, and medications come with a whole variety of potential side effects. In fact, Mary tried all sorts of pain-relieving medications, such as nonsteroidal anti-inflammatory drugs (NSAIDs) and acetaminophen, but she said they didn't work for her. Heck, she even tried morphine, and that didn't work. What could be a stronger pain-relief drug than morphine?

Even if Mary's headache pain went away because of the pain medication, once she stopped taking the pain medication, the headache would come back.

Have you ever had that experience when taking medications? When you stop taking a drug like a painkiller, muscle relaxer, or anti-inflammatory, does the pain totally go away permanently, or does it eventually come back?

It eventually comes back, doesn't it?

This is one of the drawbacks of symptom-based care that is inherent in the medical model. Symptom-based care means that the treatment focuses only on alleviating and relieving symptoms (in this case, the pain).

Even though medications may help you feel better by relieving your pain temporarily, the pain always comes back. Does this sound familiar?

Symptom-based care is predominantly centered on suppressing the expression of symptoms. It doesn't address the cause of the problem; therefore, it doesn't correct the cause of the problem, whether it's a headache, neck pain or low-back pain.

Correcting the underlying problem provides more than headache relief. After two months of chiropractic care, Mary reported that she had increased energy, improved breathing, improved bowel function, and a better ability to handle stress. But that's not all.

After twelve months of chiropractic care, Mary reported that she was more relaxed, was more restful, felt stronger, was more alert, experienced better moods, was sleeping better, noticed improved memory, experienced fewer colds and flus, was walking better, was feeling healthier, had improved digestion, and noticed her posture was improving.

Yes, her "system was restored to its natural healthy vigor." That's what health and healing is all about.

During her progress exam, in a soft-spoken but confident and cheerful voice this time, Mary told me, "Dr. Walter, I have my life back, and my health is improving. Thank you."

I love hearing those words, "thank you," but not to satisfy my ego. I love to hear them for chiropractic and for the lives that are transformed because of chiropractic. Yes, chiropractic helps with pain relief, but more than that, chiropractic helps supercharge your health, naturally, from the inside out.

Chiropractic acknowledges that your body has an innate ability to self-regulate and self-heal, which is expressed in your nervous system. Chiropractic aims to detect the interference on your nervous system and hence the interference to your body's ability to self-heal and self-regulate. The interference on the nervous system is caused by vertebral subluxations (spinal misalignments).

Chiropractic removes the interference by correcting subluxations with specific, scientific chiropractic adjustments. This restores the proper function and alignment of the spine, which allows for the innate expression of normal bodily function, healing, and repair.

There is a vast difference between
treating effects
and adjusting the cause.

—D. D. Palmer

5

Chiropractic Case Studies

Before you read the next chapter, which contains chiropractic patient stories, I want to present you with five chiropractic case studies. As you read these case studies, you will notice a common thread within them.

These are the types of health improvements that many patients experience with chiropractic care in chiropractic offices around the world.

Read on...

Case #1: Back Pain

A fifty-seven-year-old man presented with severe lower-back pain and left-leg pain that caused the patient difficulties with walking. After eight weeks of chiropractic care, the patient stated he had less back pain. Other notable improvements reported by the patient were better coordination, better emotional control, more energy, greater flexibility, improved bowel function, and a better ability to handle stress. After twelve months of chiropractic care, the patient reported feeling more relaxed, feeling more restful, being stronger, having fewer occurrences of back aches, noting improved posture, taking less medication, having more mobility, noticing better immunity, experiencing fewer colds and flus, and feeling healthier.

Case #2: Neck Pain

An eighteen-year-old woman presented with neck pain that interfered with her ability to work at her computer. The patient had suffered neck pain for three years. After eight weeks of chiropractic care, the patient reported a significant reduction in pain, from a 7 out of 10 intensity rating to a 1 out of 10 intensity rating. More than pain relief, the patient also reported feeling more relaxed, feeling more restful, sleeping better, and improved flexibility. After five months of chiropractic care, the patient stated there was no more neck pain. The patient also reported having a better mood, sleeping better, standing easier, feeling healthier, and an improvement in posture.

Case #3: Low-Back Pain and Constipation

A thirty-year-old man presented with a history of chronic constipation and low-back pain. The patient would typically have only two to three bowel movements per week. After twelve months of chiropractic care, the patient reported having no more back pain. More than pain relief, the patient also reported improved and regular daily bowel function, better emotional control, fewer colds/flus, and improved digestion.

Case #4: Pregnancy, Low-Back Pain, and Sciatica

A twenty-nine-year-old first-time mom-to-be presented with severe back pain, right-hip pain, and right sciatic leg-pain. As it was her first pregnancy, she was worried about how she would handle the pregnancy and birthing with the back and leg pain she was experiencing. The patient received chiropractic adjustments throughout her pregnancy. She experienced a reduction in back pain. Her hip pain and leg pain resolved. More than pain relief, the patient delivered her baby naturally, safely, and effortlessly during one hour of labor with no need of epidural injection, induction, or other medical interventions.

Case #5: Neck Pain, Shoulder Pain, and Numbness in Right Arm

A thirty-eight-year-old man presented with neck pain, shoulder pain, and numbness in his right arm. He was constantly fatigued and had trouble sleeping. He took pain medications and muscle relaxers but stated they only gave him temporary relief. Within eight weeks of starting chiropractic care, the patient reported a 90 percent improvement of his pain symptoms, and after ten months, he was pain free. More than pain relief, the patient also reported feeling less anxious, having greater flexibility, improved posture, feeling more relaxed and restful, having a better mood, noticing more mobility and easier walking, improvement with heartburn, improved breathing, experiencing fewer colds and flus, and better sleeping. The patient reported he was overall feeling healthier.

We celebrate all health improvements with the patients of our office. It is exhilarating to see the transformation in our patients' lives because of chiropractic care. Every day and every week we hear and see amazing patient stories. Read some of these stories now in the next chapter.

6

What Patients Are Saying about Chiropractic

One of the most rewarding aspects of being a chiropractor is seeing first-hand accounts of the transformations and health improvements patients have received from their chiropractic care.

In this chapter, you will read some of these heartfelt patient stories. They are real stories from real people. They are stories of hope, healing, and inspiration. Perhaps you will relate to some of these stories and the people who wrote them.

If you have been stressed, in pain, or suffering, as you read these stories, you will see that you are not alone. Many people share the same type of hurts and the same type of pains.

The good news is that many people have been helped with chiropractic care. As well, many people have been saved with chiropractic care.

Just know that if others can make a choice and transform their health and their life, so can you.

Special thanks go out to all the people who contributed their chiropractic patient stories to this book.

Continue to the next page to read these amazing chiropractic patient stories...

"I Hadn't Realized How Bad My Posture Was and How It Could Have Been the Reason for My Headaches"

I always had posture problems but never did anything about it. I also suffered with headaches since I was a kid and always took Tylenol because I thought it was the best "medicine". This completely changed after I had a stress-related incident at work. For about a few days, my back was in a lot of pain. I couldn't move my neck, my head felt very heavy, the light bothered me and my eyes had a burning sensation.

My mom instantly took me to see her chiropractor, mainly for my head, but for my posture too. I hadn't realized how bad my posture was and how it could have been the reason for my headaches.

Few weeks after doing chiropractic care, I started noticing that my headaches had disappeared. I never felt so good before. I stopped using painkillers.

Aside from the headaches, my health had definitely improved since I started seeing a chiropractor. I walk straighter, which makes me feel good about myself. My stress levels have gone down, and I know through this care it's helping everything else in my body.

It's like I am being healed or that my body feels more open and alive and parts are able to breathe easily.

And with that, my future is definitely brighter, and I see myself healthier. The best feeling from this is feeling the pain being relieved and washed away and that I don't have any more headaches.

Chiropractic care really changed the way I look at the body and how you're supposed to treat it, and that is what is really going to give a long life for me.

—Vivian L.

"My Body Always Felt Tense or in Pain from Either Stress or from an Injury."

Never would I have thought that receiving chiropractic care would change our family's lives for the better. My body always felt tense or in pain from either stress or from an injury.

Personally, I was experiencing stiff shoulders and neck issues plus migraines from stress and a very painful sciatic-nerve injury.

My husband, who's a plumber by trade, had a pinched nerve in his arm that would paralyze him with pain and numbness.

We were constantly at the doctor's, usually being prescribed anti-inflammatory drugs or painkillers that would mask the pain for a bit, but it would never really go away.

It wasn't until we started realigning our system through chiropractic care that we started to feel better. There was a decrease of stiffness in my neck and shoulders as well as fewer migraines. Even the pain from the sciatic nerve reduced.

My husband's numbness and discomfort in his arm practically disappeared.

We even saw a difference in our son who has autism. He became more focused and attentive at school, and his sensitivities were less disrupting.

It's now been a couple years since we started this process and we are loving how incredible we feel. Chiropractic care is a healthy lifestyle for us now, just as healthy eating and exercise are as well.

—Daniela T.

"Chiropractic Was a Choice for me Because I've Had Chronic Low-Back Pain for Years."

When I came to see the chiropractor, I had several sensations in both of my arms and legs, feet, and hands. I also suffered from anxiety due to stress and worry. It affected my life immensely. I started feeling depressed, didn't feel like working, and was on antidepressants.

Since seeing the chiropractor, I've gotten better, with the symptoms disappearing, the spine lining up properly, and my anxiety lessening. The chiropractor has educated me throughout the process and has been an unbelievable support. All his techniques are helping my spine to regenerate its health.

As time goes by with continued treatment, I am confident that I'll have a healthy life for a long time because of the chiropractor's treatments. Chiropractic was a choice for me because I've had chronic low-back pain for years. Overall, I believe chiropractic has saved me from going to a dark place.

—John F.

"The Benefits of Chiropractic Care Go a Long Way beyond Back Pain."

I have been going to a chiropractor for over eight years now. I have learned a lot of things such as how to manage back pain and stress in my life.

The benefits of chiropractic care go a long way beyond back pain. I've learned that chiropractic care is not just going to a regular checkup to fix posture and pains, but it is a way to live a long and healthy life.

—Susana S.

"On Top of All the Physical Pain, I Suffered from Chronic Anxiety, Horrible Stress, and Panic Attacks."

When I started chiropractic care five years ago it was my last hope. I was thirty years old, with two young children, and I was barely able to move. I suffered from chronic disabling back pain, daily migraines, and excruciating pain through my shoulders; my digestion was poor and my overall quality of life horrible. On top of all the physical pain, I suffered from chronic anxiety, horrible stress, and panic attacks.

Before I sought chiropractic care, I took daily Advil and other medications; I saw numerous doctors, therapists, a naturopath, and a physical therapist. I was willing to do whatever it took to get better.

At my first chiropractic consultation, I had X-rays taken to assess my condition. I remember the first time I saw my X-rays up on the screen after my chiropractic assessment. It is a feeling I will never forget. I felt like I was unfixable! As the time went on, my symptoms and pain were disappearing, and my X-rays showed that the damage was being reversed. It was amazing. I was fixable and on my way to being healed.

Since I started chiropractic care, my life has changed! I no longer have any physical pain, my migraines are gone, and I have no more anxiety or panic attacks. I believe being committed to the care plan has given me a new chance at the life I longed to have. I am active again and able to enjoy my children and family. I no longer take any medications or seek any additional therapies. I no longer suffer from anxiety, and I am able to manage my daily stress with ease.

Chiropractic is a part of my daily life, present and future, and I will continue chiropractic for myself and my children as part of a healthy lifestyle.

—Ashley L.

"I Was Suffering from Ongoing Back Aches and Headaches"

I just want to give my testimonial on how chiropractic care helped me get my overall health back on track. Before getting into any details, I would like to say that my treatments were strictly chiropractic adjustments of my spine and neck areas. There were never any new-age rituals used or any of its techniques.

I would say that I was suffering from ongoing back aches and headaches due to certain stresses, perhaps incorrect diet, and subluxations of my lower spine and neck areas. Obviously those things did not occur overnight but over some time.

Now, over the last three years that I have been receiving chiropractic care, I have seen a certain and noticeable improvement to my health from more mental clarity to physical durability and therefore less stress.

I do expect that with consistent and regular ongoing chiropractic care, my health will continue to improve.

I am happier now because I am able to do my work without the fear of falling back into pain and not receiving the proper care or treatment.

Traditional medicine just didn't do it for me; the pills and the myriad of doctor's appointments, X-rays, MRIs, and CT scans did not cut it.

Proper care and treatment are vital to health, and I found this through chiropractic care. Though I must say that conventional medicine has it place in health care, it is not the only way to go.

—Frank D.

"I Don't Want to Be Depending on Drugs to Live My Life."

I have fibromyalgia and a work injury in my upper back, neck, and shoulders. In 2007 I was diagnosed with these conditions, and I suffered with chronic pain since then.

I tried so many different treatments such as physiotherapy, massage, acoustic therapy, and much more, but I was never satisfied with the results. I am not a person who relies on medications. I don't want to be depending on drugs to live my life.

Almost a year ago, I decided to try chiropractic care, and until today I'm content that I gave it a try. Today I feel probably 75% better, I live with less pain, have more energy and better mobility. I believe I found the right treatment. My overall life improved for the better.

—Fernanda J.

"Due to My Occupation in the Construction Industry, I Find Myself Often with a Sore Neck and/or Back."

I initially started chiropractic care due to a referral on behalf of my brother-in-law who was undergoing chiropractic care. I never imagined that my spine was seriously out of alignment. I started chiropractic corrective treatment soon afterward.

Due to my occupation in the construction industry, I find myself often with a sore neck and/or back. Chiropractic care has eliminated the long-term pain that I had in my neck and back while frequent adjustments help prevent or eliminate new subluxations as they occur.

Chiropractic care has improved my overall health by reducing the effects of physical stressors that my body endures on a daily basis. I would highly recommend chiropractic care to anyone suffering pain due to misalignments. I can see myself being able to enjoy playing with my children as they grow as well as any grandchildren I may have in the future.

—Roger D.

"I Was Suffering from Severe Depression, Fibromyalgia, Chronic Lower-Back Pain, Stomach Issues, Migraines, Insomnia, and Overall My Health Was at Such a Low Point in My Life."

In life, everything happens for a reason. I had been approached throughout my life for chiropractic care. I did not consider it because I did not have an understanding of it. At a children's event, my life changed.

I was asked to have a posture assessment. At this time I was suffering from depression, fibromyalgia, chronic lower-back pain, stomach issues, migraines, insomnia, and overall my health was at such a low point in my life.

What started out as an assessment was a turning point in my life. A simple recurring plan was initialized, and quickly my symptoms began to disappear. I felt like a completely different person.

I had more energy, I slept more deeply, my back pain minimized, my migraines diminished, and my fibromyalgia disappeared.

Since I felt better physically, I started feeling better emotionally because I was not living in constant pain and struggle every day. I'm grateful that my mind was open to take this simple assessment so I could change the path in my life.

Not only does my chiropractor care for me and my family (which includes two young children), his life's mission is to heal and educate his patients to lead the healthiest life possible. We are so very lucky to have him in our lives. Our health and lives have changed forever.

—Rosie N.

"I Felt Like My Body Was Ruined and I Would Never Walk without a Limp Or Climb Stairs without Pain."

Chiropractic changed my life. After I left the army, I felt like my body was ruined and I would never walk without a limp or climb stairs without pain. I am so glad I was wrong!

Under chiropractic care for the last two years, I have given birth to two healthy babies, and I feel as a young as I did before I joined the military. Chiropractic care has undone those years of bodily abuse and restored me to a place where I don't regret my years of service. I look forward to many future active years keeping up with my children without fear of stairs or knee or hip-replacement surgery.

Our whole family is hooked on chiropractic care now. Our youngest child was adjusted three days after birth to reverse birth trauma, and we all have regular adjustments because we've seen and felt the benefits of a well-aligned spine—physically, emotionally and health-wise as well.

—**Mindy D.**

"I Suffered with Pain and Discomfort through My Twenties Going into My Thirties."

Before chiropractic care I was always in pain and discomfort in my upper back and neck. I thought there was something wrong with my muscle. I suffered with pain and discomfort through my twenties going into my thirties.

I would try to crack my neck practically daily to get some relief, but it didn't help. I started chiropractic care three to four years ago. After just a few adjustments, I immediately started to feel pain relief and felt more mobile.

Little did I know that the pain was due to the alignment of my spine. Chiropractic care had done a world of difference for me. I am pain free and loving it.

I will continue with chiropractic care. It is great for your well-being and pain relief. I highly recommend chiropractic care to anyone.

—very happy patient, **Sandy M.**

"It Was Very Easy to Take Painkillers to Get Rid of the Pain for Temporary Relief, But It Was Not Lasting."

I have played many sports growing up and have taken a few bumps along the way. As a youngster I didn't have the knowledge or experience to know that I should have had these "bumps" (now I call them subluxations) looked at.

When I was forty-six years old, I was feeling it in the joints when getting out of bed. It was easy to take painkillers to get rid of the pain for temporary relief, but it was not lasting, and I was not sure what other damage the drugs caused.

I met my chiropractor over one year ago, and he taught me about back to health the chiropractic way and how to cure the root cause of pain and treat it, not hide it with painkillers.

I am no longer feeling the pain. I am less stressed and able to concentrate more. Overall, I am feeling great. Power's up!

—Gianluca S.

"I Didn't Come to the Chiropractic Office with Any Specific Symptoms or Health Issues Other than a General Desire to Be Healthy."

I started seeing the chiropractor several years ago. I didn't come to the chiropractic office with any specific symptoms or health issues other than a general desire to be healthy.

The chiropractic work I had was, I felt, relatively routine—traction and adjustments to correct a foreword neck posture, very common—and, with treatment, it's corrected and being maintained.

What I didn't expect was the overall positive effect visiting the chiropractor has had on my general health and well-being. His workshops, ranging from stress relief to nutrition to healthy pregnancies, really appealed to me, and it was through these that I saw the most positive change. His encouraging attitude and leading by example doesn't hurt, either.

I was hoping to lose weight two to three years ago, and my chiropractor had a good lending library. I found a book that spoke to me about food in the right way, and this changed how I approached my diet.

At the time I didn't exercise enough and just changed how I ate, and through this and my chiropractor's encouragement, maintained a lifestyle change that led to dropping (and keeping off) twenty-five to thirty pounds.

I appreciated that he has a quality scale that not only monitors weight but also fat percentage, and monthly measuring allowed me to monitor progress even when I didn't physically see any.

I also made an effort to join his run/walk club, and through the supportive attitudes of all attending, I was inspired to keep training on my own, noticing improvement over the summer. I used a running program app and was thrilled each time I went to the run/walk club that I could go further than the session before. I've since completed a few 5Ks within my goal time—beating a time I had from nearly ten years ago!

Now, I'm currently approximately eight months into my first pregnancy. I have continued to see my chiropractor every two weeks. While every pregnancy is different, I've noticed that mine was comparatively easy thus far—no morning sickness, few symptoms, and minor back pain...much less than many other women at this stage. I credit my overall health and my chiropractic visits.

Thanks to the resources at my chiropractor's center and my chiropractor's belief in the body's abilities, I also feel that my body is fully capable of managing delivery in a very positive way. Regular chiropractic is also supposed to decrease labor time and pain. I'll find out soon enough!

I never expected to receive the support and encouragement to make such lifestyle changes from a chiropractor. My chiropractor really is obviously invested in the overall health and well-being of his patients, and it's what keeps us coming back.

We moved to a different town two years ago, and we still make the visits. I'll not be able to forget the immensely positive effect my chiropractor has had on not only my life, but that of my family's, and for that I am grateful.

—**Erica P.**

We get sick because of something inside going wrong! We get well because of something inside going right!

—B. J. Palmer

7

The Stress Burden

Did you have any stress in your life this past month? What about this past week? How about today?

I am finding that almost every single patient who walks through my front door, regardless of their age, is stressed out.

For instance, Mary told me that she was often stressed out. She had trouble coping with her work because she had constant pounding headaches. She was an account manager, and her work required her to sit in front of a computer all day. She was busy at work and often overwhelmed with deadlines.

She loved her family time but was unhappy because her headaches prevented her from spending quality time with her children and husband. Her downtime after work involved resting in a dark, quiet room hoping for her pounding headache to subside so she could get back to spending time with her children and husband.

Just like Mary, everyone else experiences stress. Even children experience stress. One day, a mom brought in her six-year-old daughter for a spinal checkup. The mom told me her daughter had digestive problems and constipation. The mom also told me that her daughter was a high achiever in school and a perfectionist who got extremely upset when she made mistakes with her schoolwork. You see, children experience stress, too.

Teenagers also experience stress. For instance, in high school, bullying is a serious cause of emotional stress for many teenagers. Also, heavy backpacks, the use of multimedia devices, and slouching are common sources of physical stress in teens, causing bad posture to develop.

For adults, stress comes from all sorts of life situations like work, finances, and relationship problems. Sounds familiar?

But what is stress, and how does it affect your life and your health?

Have you ever experienced something like this? You find yourself in a stressful situation—perhaps you were involved in a sudden and unexpected car accident, perhaps you had an argument with a coworker, or perhaps you had a worrisome thought about a particular circumstance in your life.

Your heart begins to race. You can feel your heart pounding in your chest. You begin to sweat. You feel hot. Your breathing changes; you're breathing faster. Your muscles tense, and you have butterflies in your stomach.

What you just read describes the changes, reactions and responses your body goes through when you are under stress. This response is called the fight-or-flight response.

The Fight-or-Flight Response

The fight-or-flight response is a natural physiologic response that is designed to enable you to run away from or fight off a threatening situation.

This response occurs every time you encounter or experience a stressful situation. The stressful situation can be real, like a car accident that just occurred, or it can be imagined, like worrying about something that has not yet happened.

Each time you experience or perceive a threat or stress, your brain, through a system of hormonal glands, begins a process of releasing stress hormones into your bloodstream.

These stress hormones are called adrenaline (epinephrine) and cortisol. Stress hormones trigger all the bodily changes associated with the fight-or-flight response.

This type of fight-or-flight response would have been extremely useful in primitive times when early humans were facing threats from wild animals or attacks from neighboring tribes.

Of course, if you were out on a nature hike today and you encountered a bear, the fight-or-flight response would be very useful so you could run away or try to fight it off to save yourself.

⌘

The fight-or-flight response is designed to be short-lived.

But in today's modern society, we are not typically faced with these types of stresses or threats. You may not encounter a bear today, but you may be stressed because of work.

Regardless of the source of stress, whether it's real or imagined, your bodily response is the exact same—the release of stress hormones and the initiation of the fight-or-flight response.

Here is a key point about the fight-or-flight response. The fight-or-flight response and the subsequent release of the stress hormones (adrenaline and cortisol) are designed to be short-lived.

That is, the stress response in your body was designed for you to deal with the immediate threat (the stressor) so that you could run away from it or fight it off. It's a survival mechanism meant to be used for an instance of a few minutes.

This is how it works. Let's say you encounter a bear on your nature hike, your fight-or-flight response kicks in, the stress hormones are released, your heart rate increases, blood rushes to your legs and other muscles, and your muscles tense up.

You prepare to protect yourself (fight) or run away from the bear (flight). Once the bear (the stressor) is gone, the fight-or-flight response stops, the stress hormones are no longer released, and your body systems returns to their balanced state.

But what if the bear does not go away? In other words, what if the stress was always there? Then you would constantly be in a fight-or-flight response.

> ⌘
>
> **Stress can come from trauma, toxins, or thoughts.**

You would constantly have the stress hormones, adrenaline and cortisol, releasing in your bloodstream. And your body would constantly be experiencing the effects of the fight-or-flight response— the increased blood pressure, increased heart rate, and increased muscle tension.

Also, other important bodily functions and systems would be inhibited, such as digestion, immunity, reproduction and tissue healing because these systems are not required during a stressful fight-or-flight situation.

While you are not likely to encounter stress from a bear in your day-to-day living, you are, however, likely to encounter a stressor that repeats regularly and eventually turns into a persistent chronic stress.

Stress can come from these three main categories:

1. Physical stresses (traumas)
2. Chemical stresses (toxins)
3. Emotional stresses (thoughts)

Here are some common forms of stress people experience for each of these categories:

Physical Stresses (Trauma)

- Bad posture
- Sitting in front of a computer/laptop
- Using handheld devices like smartphones, tablets, video games
- Bad sleeping positions
- Working in awkward positions
- Repetitive movements
- Falls, accidents, sports
- Birth trauma
- Improper lifting

Chemical Stresses (Toxins)

- Drugs (prescription, over-the-counter, street)
- Smoking
- Alcohol
- Caffeine (coffee, soda pop)
- Environmental pollutants
- Household-cleaning solvents and solutions
- Food additives, preservatives, and colors
- Sugar, sweeteners, corn syrup

Emotional Stresses (Thoughts)

- Work, overwhelming deadlines
- Worry about paying bills, finances
- Illness, disease, dying
- Disputes and disagreements with loved ones (parents, siblings, spouses, children, friends)
- Negative self-talk
- Divorce
- Anger, fear, worry, anxiety, guilt
- Unresolved emotional hurts
- Bullying

Can you see how, in your day-to-day life, you can be exposed to stressful scenarios and situations from multiple sources?

Now what if your stress is always there? What if you are always stressed out, day in and day out? And what if you don't have coping strategies to effectively conquer your stress?

If you experience one, two, or several of the these stresses on a regular daily basis, your stress response will always be turned on, and it will eventually become chronic.

For many people, chronic stress seems to be an ongoing and inevitable part of their life. When not handled effectively, stress, and eventually chronic stress, can become a detriment to your health.

Chronic stress has been associated with insomnia, muscle pain, high blood pressure, a weakened immune system, heart disease, obesity, anxiety, and depression.[1]

Ongoing Stress → Chronic Stress → Disease

When stress is chronic in your life, when the stress is always there, your brain will always initiate the fight-or-flight response, and there will always be a release of stress hormones in your body. This will occur regardless of what the source of stress is for you.

The source of stress can be from a physical, chemical, or emotional source. The source of stress is totally irrelevant to your brain—the fight-or-flight response will always be triggered. The burden of stress is detrimental to your health and can lead to serious health problems.

> ⌘
>
> **Ongoing stress is detrimental to your health and can lead to serious health problems.**

If there is one thing you can be certain about with stress, it is this—stress will always show up in life. At some point in your life, you will have stress. At some point in your life, you will be stressed out.

The key is to learn how to manage your stress so it doesn't cause ongoing health problems. One essential strategy to conquering stress is chiropractic care. One of the key benefits I have consistently seen people get from chiropractic care is a better ability to handle stress. Read on to discover how.

8

Conquering the Stress Burden with Chiropractic

So many people are stressed out these days. Some people are more stressed out than others.

Consider that a 2013 *Canadian Community Health Survey* by Statistics Canada found that 23 percent of Canadians aged fifteen and older reported that most days were "extremely stressful" or "quite a bit stressful."[1] This survey also reported that daily stress rates were highest in the core working ages of thirty-five to fifty-four.

Similarly, a 2013 report entitled *Stress in America,* by the American Psychological Association, revealed that 36 percent of American adults surveyed reported feeling more stress compared to the previous year.[2] This report also showed that 31 percent of American teens reported their stress increased compared to the previous year.

Why is stress so prevalent today? Why is perceived stress on the rise?

A lot has to do with how busy people are these days. People lead busy lives. They are overwhelmed at work, and they are busy with family life. Many parents have their children in multiple after-school programs that keep them on the go after work with little down time for rest and recovery. This overwhelming after-school schedule can be very stressful to parents.

As for children and teens, they experience stress at home and also at school. Consider, too, the increased exposure children and teens have to entertainment multimedia inputs coming from television, Internet, social media sites, video games, DVD players, mp3 players, smartphones, and tablet devices.

A 2010 study by The Henry J. Kaiser Family Foundation reported that third- through twelfth-grade students (aged eight to eighteen) spend on average seven hours and thirty-eight minutes a day using entertainment media.[3] This adds up to more than fifty-three hours a week.

The ergonomic stress with this much use of entertainment media cannot be overlooked. When using these media devices, children and teens do not usually sit in the optimal posture or position to minimize strain or stress on the spine and muscles.

They end up slouching and shifting their heads forward while playing games, surfing the net, or texting on their smartphones. And oftentimes, they are playing or using their computers for hours at a time without getting up. The consequence for children and teens is that the spine and posture get stressed and misaligned over time.

People are so busy that they make little time for simple things like going for a walk in nature, exercising, reading a good book, or having quality conversations with family and friends. In some cases, the only recovery time people get is a one-week vacation, once or twice a year, only to come back to the daily grind of life, both at work and home. And many people don't even take vacations or give themselves recovery time, so they never break up their stress patterns.

> ⌘
>
> **A forward head position causes tension on the spinal cord, which causes interference on your nervous system.**

Add to that, the physical stress you are exposed to on a daily basis at work. Do you sit all day at a computer desk? This is a primary source of physical stress. Slouching in the chair will lead to a forward head position. A forward head places undue stress on the spinal bones of your neck and it causes muscle tension in your neck, shoulders, and upper back. A forward head position also causes tension on the spinal cord, which causes interference on your nervous system.

Some jobs require physical labor and working in awkward positions. Other jobs involve repetitive bending and lifting. These are other common sources of physical stress.

Physical stress can also come from bad sleeping positions. The best way to sleep is on your back or on your side because this supports the natural curves of your spine. Sleeping on your stomach is not recommended and must be avoided.

When you sleep on your stomach, your head and neck will always be turned to one side because you have to allow for an open airway for breathing. Having your neck turned and tilted up on a pillow while you are sleeping on your stomach throughout the night will certainly add stress to the spinal bones, spinal nerves, and muscles of your neck.

> ⌘
>
> **A negative emotional state is a predominant source of stress.**

Physical stresses can also be caused from accidents, falls, and sporting injuries. These types of traumas are usually sudden, hard, and fast and definitely cause stress to your body, especially to the spine.

With some patients, I have noticed that a negative emotional state is their predominant source of stress, especially negative self-talk. Having a negative and unsupportive belief system is unhealthy. Examples of negative self-talk are statements like, "I'm not good enough," "I'm such an idiot," "I hate myself," and "No one loves me."

Negative emotional states, such as low self-esteem and low confidence, can cause someone to slouch forward as a protective mechanism, leading to bad posture over time and stress on the spine, nerves, and spinal cord. Buried negative emotional experiences from years past or from childhood are a common source of hidden stress.

Then there are chemical stresses. Chemicals in the food, air, and water are toxic to the body and organ systems and place them under stress. Take a look at some food and beverage labels to see how many of the ingredients consist of preservatives, colors, flavor enhancers, sweeteners, and other artificial additives.

What about the household cleaners and solvents that you may be using? Most commonly used cleaning solutions are toxic and poisonous. If you live in the city or a suburb, the quality of the air is not as clean as it would be out in the countryside. Chemicals and toxins from all these sources can cause sensitivities and stimulate the stress response in your body.

Day in and day out, stress places a burden on your body and on your nervous system. When you are constantly exposed to stress, there is a constant secretion of cortisol in your body that activates the sympathetic nervous system. The sympathetic nervous system is part of the autonomic nervous system, which controls the fight-or-flight response of your body.

Stress Activates the Fight-or-Flight Part of Your Nervous System

When the sympathetic nervous system is activated by stress, it increases heart rate and blood pressure, it increases blood-sugar levels, and it tenses muscles. All this occurs in response to a stressful situation to prepare you for fight-or-flight.

If the stressful situation persists without effective coping strategies, it can lead to chronic stress. Chronic stress burdens and overloads the sympathetic nervous system. When you are constantly stressed out, you are essentially in sympathetic nervous system overdrive. Chronic stress leads to chronic diseases, such as high blood pressure, heart disease, anxiety and obesity.

Stress Inhibits Organs That Are Not Needed During the Fight-or-Flight Response

It's important to note that organ systems that are not essential to a fight-or-flight situation will be inhibited, such as the digestive system, the immune system, and the reproductive system.

These organ systems are controlled by the parasympathetic nervous system, which is also part of the autonomic nervous system.

This may explain why people who are constantly stressed out are more susceptible to colds, flus, infections, illness, fertility problems, and digestive disorders like constipation, diarrhea, and colitis.

Stress can place a burden on your quality of life, your quality of health, your happiness, your peace of mind, and your overall well-being.

It is therefore essential that you have effective stress-coping strategies or a solid stress-management plan. Unfortunately, in most cases, you cannot predict when the next stressful situation will occur, but if you have a readiness plan for managing the stress when it does appear, you will be well equipped to conquer that stress so you can live a more enjoyable and peaceful life.

Although many people come to the chiropractic office seeking pain relief, one of the biggest benefits people get from regular chiropractic care is a better ability to handle stress. For anyone who is sick, suffering from pain, or simply stressed out, chiropractic care is a viable option not only for natural relief of pain but also to promote a healthier quality of life.

Chiropractic's aim is to detect and correct vertebral subluxations. Stress from any source, whether it be physical, chemical, or emotional, will always trigger stress hormones to be released, initiating the fight-or-flight response in your body. As part of the fight-or-flight response, muscles become tense.

> ⌘
> **Chiropractic's aim is to detect and correct vertebral subluxations.**

Stress and Muscle Tension

Muscle tension, primarily along the spinal column in the neck, upper back, mid-back, and lower back, will cause restrictions in the normal motion and function of the spinal bones. Said another way, stress will cause vertebral subluxations to develop.

Stress and Bad Posture

Stress also causes bad posture to develop. When the body is under stress, the brain sends out a protective response that causes your posture to curl and slouch forward, similar to the fetal position. Getting into the fetal position always feels comforting and protective. However, when it occurs in a prolonged state, it causes bad posture, such as rounded shoulders and a forward head position.

Posture displacements like these over a prolonged time become set in those positions, causing global subluxations in the spine. A global subluxation means that several spinal bones in a row become shifted away from optimal position. Whether subluxations occur in one, two, or a series of spinal bones, they will cause tension on the nerves and spinal cord.

Recall that the nervous system controls all bodily functions, all healing, and all tissue repairs. Tension on the nerves and spinal cord from subluxations will interfere with the vital connection between brain and body.

This means subluxations will interfere with the optimal function of your organ systems, your innate healing potential, and your body's tissue repair mechanism. You cannot express full health when you have vertebral subluxations because your body's innate ability to function, heal, and repair is compromised.

Vertebral Subluxations Must Be Corrected

Several key things happen when vertebral subluxations are corrected with chiropractic adjustments. The motion and function of the spinal bones improve. This means less muscle tension and more mobility. Improved spinal motion leads to less strain and stress on the tissue of the spine, ligaments, tendons, muscles, and discs.

These tissues are very sensitive to pain, and when they are strained and stressed by subluxations, inflammation and pain result. Chiropractic adjustments improve the normal function and motion of the spinal bones; this corrects subluxations and optimizes the spinal function and structure, thereby relieving the strain and stress on the pain-sensitive ligaments, tendons, muscles, and discs. The result is pain relief.

Chiropractic care offers a unique and natural approach to pain relief by correcting the cause of the underlying pain condition. In many cases, the cause of the underlying pain condition is subluxations of the spine.

Of course, the only way to determine if subluxations are causing your pain condition is by getting a spinal exam with a chiropractor. Chiropractors are the go-to-experts for detecting and correcting vertebral subluxations.

Recall that when the stress response is initiated in your body, cortisol hormone is secreted. Cortisol activates the sympathetic nervous system organs and functions while inhibiting the parasympathetic nervous system organs and functions.

The parasympathetic nervous system is mostly activated at rest and is often called the "rest and digest" system. If the sympathetic nervous system is chronically activated by daily stresses and the parasympathetic nervous system is consequently chronically inhibited, this poses a serious imbalance in your bodily systems.

Recall, too, that your body always wants to remain at homeostasis, in constant balance. One of the key benefits of chiropractic care is that spinal adjustments help to bring balance back to the sympathetic nervous system and the parasympathetic nervous system.

Chiropractic adjustments in key areas of the spine will help stimulate the parasympathetic nervous system. This helps counteract the sympathetic nervous system overload and therefore minimize the stress response in the body.

The result is a better ability to handle and conquer stress when a stress scenario appears.

As for Mary, she was a woman who was in pain, was suffering, and stressed out, and she has completely turned her life around. In fact, she had a transformation. She became happier, healthier, and free of headaches and now enjoys a better quality of life with her family.

It all started with a choice, a choice for healing. And her healing and transformation came to fruition because of her strong commitment and follow through.

But how long would Mary carry on and follow through with her choice for better health and a better quality of life? Again, this is one of those important questions that I never know the answer to because it's always up to the patient.

However, I have noticed that patients who create a long-lasting life vision for themselves, have the strongest commitment and follow through to lifelong health and wellness.

9

Casting a Vision
for Your Life

What is vision? At my clinic, I talk about vision during our new patient orientation class and seminars. When I speak about vision in the context of your life, I am not talking about the act of sensing or seeing with your eyes. Not that kind of vision.

When I speak about vision I am specifically talking about casting a picture of what you want your life to look like in the future. Some people have a clear vision of how they want their life to be, but a majority of people do not.

Your life purpose, your happiness, your health, your peace of mind, and your quality of life moving forward into the future are a function of how clear your life vision looks to you now. Read that last sentence again.

I always like to refer to a dictionary to discover the root meaning of words. If you look up the word *vision*, you will see about seven different definitions. The one that is most appropriate for this discussion is this: "Vision: a vivid, imaginative conception or anticipation."[1]

A vision for your life is a vivid conception. A vision for your life is imaginative. In other words, it's a mental picture of how you want your life to be. The vision of your life is conceived—it's formed by you. The vision of your life is anticipated—it's something you expect in advance. You can create any vision for your life, but it's you who must create it.

At my clinic, our mission is this:

To help sick and suffering people get well with chiropractic care so they can live a long-lasting, healthy, and happy life.

What drives our team to fulfill this mission is our vision statement. We are inspired daily by the vision we hold for our patients. Our vision statement creates a context for which our patients can create a vision for themselves.

Creating a vision for your life is precious. When you are clear on the direction you are heading in your life, where you want to be in the next twenty, thirty, forty, fifty, sixty, seventy years, you begin to make the appropriate choices today that will lead you into your vision.

James Allen, in his masterpiece book, "*As a Man Thinketh*" says this about vision: "He who cherishes a beautiful vision, a lofty ideal in his heart, will one day realize it."2

He also says this...

Dream lofty dreams, and as you dream, so shall you become. Your Vision is the promise of what you shall one day be; your Ideal is the prophecy of what you shall at last unveil.

You literally step into your vision every single day with each choice you make on a daily basis. And that's a powerful way to live.

You may already have a vision for your life. That's great. Go with it, and continue doing the positive things today that will help you fulfill your vision down the road.

If you don't know your life vision, that's OK right now. But make it a goal to create and cast the ideal vision for yourself and your life, one that you fully desire to live into. Start working on your vision today.

Some suggestions could be to create an ideal image for your family life/relationship, your career/business, your health, your recreation, and your finances.

It helps to clip out pictures and images from magazines or from the Internet and post them on a board. This vision board serves as a constant visual reminder of your ideal life vision.

Now, let's bring this all together. If you were to ask me, "Dr. Walter, how can I make a lasting change with my health and well-being?" I would answer with these three words—"Vision. Choices. Commitment."

Back To Health Chiropractic Centre's Vision Statement

Children, youths, and families realizing their full potential, living with the full expression of health and love, enjoying a long-lasting, healthy, happy, and active quality of life.

CHILDREN who are growing healthy and strong, living into their full human potential.

YOUTHS who are following their life vision and fulfilling their life dreams.

FAMILIES who are flourishing, healthy, and happy.

PATIENTS who are creating miracles and experiencing love, joy, and peace—in their lives, in their families, and in their relationships. Patients who are healing naturally, being healthy, staying healthy.

LONG-LASTING, HEALTHY, HAPPY, AND ACTIVE QUALITY OF LIFE
Our vision is that all our patients are healthy, whole, and complete—physically, mentally, emotionally, and spiritually.

We are committed to the fulfilment of this vision. We are committed that all our patients—all children, youths, and families—live an extraordinary life of health, love, and happiness.

Vision: Know what you want and why.

Choices: Make the choices that are aligned with your life vision.

Commitment: Commit yourself to do whatever it takes to achieve your vision.

To illustrate how vision, choices, and commitment are intertwined, I will share with you my first marathon experience. I ran my first full marathon in Toronto in 2009.

⌘

Vision will guide your life direction and your life choices.

The day before the race, I went to pick up my race packet at the expo, and I began looking at some pictures of past marathon runners. I was impressed to see a picture of a ninety-year-old man running that exact same marathon in the past. Yes! Ninety-years-old and he ran 42.2 kilometers. Imagine that! It was thrilling to know that he accomplished it.

That's when I said, "One day, when I'm ninety years old, I shall do the same and run a marathon."

In that moment, I created a vision for my life for the next fifty-plus years that would dictate the lifestyle choices I would make today; these will be the lifestyle choices that support the fulfillment of my vision.

At the instant when I made that declaration, my mind started racing. I started asking questions like this, *What do I have to start doing today to help me reach ninety years of age and be physically fit to run a marathon?*

My choices instantly became clear. Exercise and run regularly. Eat wholesome, nutritious foods. Keep an ideal body weight. Keep my spine healthy and optimized with chiropractic care. I realized I would have to start making choices today consistent with my vision to accomplish that dream.

> ⌘
>
> **Your quality of life and your quality of health depend on you and the choices you make.**

I also realized that a strong commitment and follow through every step of the way were essential requirements. This is the power of vision. Vision will guide your life direction and your life choices.

Let me ask you this: What is your vision, and what is the "why" behind your vision? How will you choose in the face of tempting and conflicting options or opportunities that may steer you off course? Are you prepared to commit yourself and do whatever it takes to fulfill that vision?

When it comes to your health, your relationships, your family, your job, or whatever else is of value to you, create a clear vision of how you want it to look. Always make choices in the direction of your vision and commit yourself to achieving your vision.

Your quality of life and your quality of health depend on you and the choices you make. When you have a clear vision for your life, you will make choices that are congruent and aligned with your ideal life vision.

I realize that most people who walk into my office for the first time don't have a clear, long-lasting vision for their life. Some patients are initially only looking for immediate relief of their pain and immediate resolution of their symptoms.

For some people, their vision is for short-term relief, and so their choices only take them on to the point of pain relief. But being without pain or symptoms does not mean you are healthy.

The World Health Organization (WHO) defines health like this: "Health is a state of complete physical, mental and social well-being and not merely the absence of disease or infirmity."[3]

In my chiropractic practice, the vision statement is the foundation. My intention is to lead and guide our patients to create their own vision for their life so they can truly experience a long-lasting, healthy, active, and happy life that is unique to them and their own ideals.

For that to happen, they must make a choice for healing because healing is for the long run versus for immediate relief.

Mary was looking for relief of her headaches. That's what brought her to my chiropractic office. But when she made a choice for healing, her life started to transform. Mary attended many of our wellness seminars and also participated in our run/walk club.

She started eating better, she began exercising, and she developed strategies for managing her stress. I realized she created a new, healthier vision for her life, and her new actions reflected that vision. The new lifestyle choices she was making as she continued on with her chiropractic care were aligned with the new vision of her life.

What would be the result for someone who is chronically overweight, smokes, has a poor diet, is lazy, gets no exercise, and is constantly under stress with no effective stress-management strategies? It doesn't require a doctor's degree to know that there is a high probability this person will end up sick, have a poor quality of life, and possibly die well before his or her potential life expectancy. Does that make sense?

Now, in contrast, if someone keeps an ideal body weight; exercises regularly; eats good, wholesome, nutritious foods; has effective management strategies for their stress; and has a clear, compelling vision for his or her life, this person would most likely live a complete life, full of energy, health, and vitality. Wouldn't they?

Well, many people have already been told that it's important to eat well, exercise regularly, and find ways to manage stress. You may have even heard the same advice.

However, have you ever been told to keep your spine optimized, free of subluxations? Probably not, unless you've been to a chiropractic office like ours that teaches this to you.

This is why chiropractic care has been called the missing piece of the puzzle. I say chiropractic care is the missing piece of the *health-care* puzzle.

Your nervous system controls all your bodily functions, all your muscle movements and coordination, all your healing, and all your bodily repair mechanisms. You experience your environment and your life through your nervous system—touch, smell, taste, hearing, seeing, movement, concentration, learning, memory, talking, emotions, behaviour, and communication.

To express full health and full potential, you need a healthy nervous system that is free of interference. So it's imperative that the spine, which houses the spinal cord, be free of subluxations. An optimal spine means optimal health.

Today, many people living in rich, industrialized countries like Canada and the United States resort first to taking medications. Our society has become a population of overmedicated citizens.

According to the National Center of Health Statistics, prescription drug use by Americans has increased, from about 39 percent of Americans taking prescription drugs in 1988-1994 to about 47 percent in 2007-2010.[4] The percentage of Americans taking five or more drugs also increased from 4 percent in 1988-1994 to about 10 percent in 2007-2010.

People take all sorts of medications just to cope with their pain, or as a treatment for their health problem.

I had one patient tell me she took seven painkillers for her headache just so she can get through the day.

Another woman showed me her list of medicines; it listed twelve drugs. Everyday she was taking drugs for pain, inflammation, high cholesterol, high blood pressure, stomach and thyroid problems.

There was this ten-year-old boy whose mom told me he was prescribed eight prednisone pills a day for colitis.

That is an enormous amount of drugs that are being taken. Do you agree?

If prescription drug use is increasing, are people getting healthier? The short answer is *no!*

A 2010 report by Statistics Canada called *Fitness of Canadian Adults: Results from the 2007-2009 Canadian Health Measures Survey*, examined the fitness levels of Canadians.[5] This study found that there has been a decrease in muscular strength, a decrease in flexibility and an increase in obesity in Canadians since 1981, all of which can pose significant health risks.

More prescription drugs are being taken but people are getting sicker, not healthier.

If that doesn't disturb you, check this out...

The UNICEF Office of Research–Innocenti published a report in 2013 called *Child Well-Being in Rich Countries: A Comparative Overview*, which measured and compared the well-being children have achieved in the world's richest nations.[6] Here are some shocking findings...

Canada ranks in a middle position, at seventeen of twenty-nine nations, for the overall well-being of its children. With regards to the health and safety of its children, Canada ranks at twenty-seven of twenty-nine industrialized countries. For infant mortality, Canada ranks twenty-second.

As for the United States, it ranks twenty-sixth of twenty-nine in the overall well-being of its children. For the health and safety of its children, the United States ranks twenty-fifth, and for infant mortality it ranks twenty-sixth.

So, let me ask you ... Where are the health and welfare of our children and our society heading when more drugs are being prescribed these days yet people are getting sicker, not healthier?

You see, more medicines, more drugs, more pills is not the answer to personal health care. I am not discounting the use of medications during a health crisis, such as a deadly bacterial infection, or during an emergency, such as a serious life-threatening injury.

However, for the common, daily ailments and pain conditions people experience day in and day out, drugs may not always be the answer to correcting the underlying problem.

No amount of drugs permanently cleared Mary's headaches, not even morphine, one of the strongest pain-relief drugs. That's because health does not come from a bottle of chemicals. There is no such thing as better living with chemistry. It's about better living through better, healthier lifestyle choices.

> ⌘
>
> **More medicines, more drugs, more pills is *not* the answer to personal health care.**

To create a transformation in your health and your life, you must start making better, healthier lifestyle choices. A healthy lifestyle is a decision away.

The common health problems that plague many people today, such as heart disease, cancer, diabetes, and obesity, are often preventable diseases. This means that, oftentimes, these conditions develop because of things that we do to ourselves on a daily basis.

Your lifestyle choices are a big deal when it comes to enjoying your best health. Your lifestyle choices are a big deal, too, when it comes to preventing heart disease, cancer, diabetes, and obesity.

You see, being healthy is a decision away. What this means is that you have the power to be healthy, stay healthy, or get healthy. It starts with a decision, such as: "I am committing to being the healthiest I can be, now and forever".

> ⌘
>
> **Your lifestyle choices are a big deal when it comes to enjoying your best health.**

Say this out loud now in the form of a declaration. A declaration is a positive affirmation stated out loud. Stand up right now, put your hand on your heart, and say out loud:

"I am committing to being the healthiest I can be, now and forever."

If you didn't do it, ask yourself why. That will be your lesson here. How serious can you be about your health if you cannot make this simple declaration right now?

It's your choice, isn't it? Life is about choices, yes? And so is your health.

Stand up and commit to your health today, now and forever!

"I am committing to being the healthiest I can be, now and forever."

How did that feel?

Say this declaration every morning when you wake up and every night before you go to bed. Do it for the next thirty days and watch how your life and your health will transform.

Next, write down your health goals and what your ideal life vision is for the next thirty-plus years.

Always write your goals and vision in the present tense. Writing is a powerful way to get your ideas from thought form into a more tangible form that you can see. An example of a health goal is, "I am exercising three hours per week." Another example is, "I now weigh 158 pounds." Keep the paper with your goals and vision with you at all times in your pocket or purse because if it's out of sight, it's out of mind.

> ⌘
>
> **Being healthy, staying healthy or getting healthy is a choice.**

Next, commit to making the lifestyle choices that are aligned with and that will move you closer to your goals and ideal life vision. Being healthy, staying healthy, or getting healthy is a choice. The choice is yours.

With that, other choices follow that will keep you on the path of wellness and health.

Good choices involve eating nutritious foods, exercising regularly every week, managing your stress with effective coping strategies, planning for your life with inspiring goals, and regular chiropractic care to keep your spine and nervous system healthy.

I call it the **5 Pillars of Great Health**:

1. Healthy Spine and Nervous System
2. Stress Management
3. Nutrition
4. Exercise
5. Vision, Purpose, and Life Goals

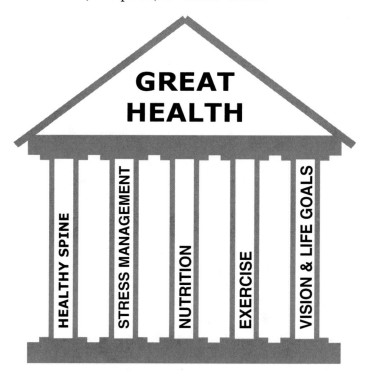

In my office, I teach a seminar series in each of the **5 Pillars of Great Health**. Through our seminars, we lead and guide our patients to make healthier lifestyle choices so they can live a long-lasting, healthy, happy, and active life.

You too must be making lifestyle choices in all these **5 Pillars of Great Health** for you to create a solid foundation for a vibrant life.

Yes, a healthy, happy, peaceful, stronger, and energetic life is a lifestyle. This lifestyle requires a choice, a decision made with intent.

Are you up to making that decision today for a healthy lifestyle? It starts with you.

You have the power to choose. You have the power to heal. You have all the answers within you.

Sometimes, all that is needed is a little guidance...a little nudge. So choose powerfully. Choose wisely. Seek guidance when needed. And always make your choices in line with the ideal vision of your life. Remember to commit to making these favorable, supportive lifestyle choices.

To keep on track with making these choices consistently, you must have a clear, compelling vision for your life. With a clear, compelling vision for your life, you will always make clear-cut choices that are aligned with your ideal vision.

For millions of people, chiropractic care represents a choice. It's a choice for a natural form of pain relief. But more than that, it's a choice for healing. With that comes the transformation into a long-lasting, healthy, happy, and active life.

If you are in pain, have been suffering, are stressed out, and are looking to supercharge your health, give chiropractic a try. Visit a chiropractic office in your community. Chiropractic may very well be the missing piece of your personal health-care puzzle.

If you are already seeing a chiropractor, congratulations! You have made a wise choice for your healing, for your health care, and for the future vision of your life. Keep it going! Keep up your commitment to your health, and follow through with your chiropractic care.

10

Back to Health by Choice the Chiropractic Way

Being healthy and staying healthy require a conscious choice, as well as a commitment and a long-range vision for your life.

No one should care more about your health and your life than you. Which means you need to first take care of number one, and that's you!

You are important. You are worthy. Before you can take care of the people in your life, you need to be energetic, strong, and healthy yourself. Do you agree? You need to be taking care of yourself.

If you are sick, if you are suffering from any ailments, or if you are in constant pain, take a stand today for creating a transformation in your health and in your life.

Every human is in search of happiness. Life is about living out your full human potential. That's what creates ultimate happiness—knowing you discovered your purpose and are living your ideal life vision.

Even if you are sick, suffering, or in pain, you can still take control of your life. You have power over your thoughts. You have power over your choices.

So if you are sick, suffering, stressed out, or in pain, and you want to create a transformation in your health and in your life, you must make a choice to get back to health.

Do not lose hope!

You read a lot about choice in this book. Do not underestimate the power to choose that which you desire.

This book is about a choice for healing. There is power in intention. The answers will come your way when you make a choice for healing and you commit to your choice.

As I mentioned earlier, chiropractic represents a form of healing that many people can accept based on their values, beliefs, and paradigms. If chiropractic resonates with you, give chiropractic a try.

Chiropractic is one form of healing with a unique approach that makes sense to a lot of people who choose it. Millions of people choose chiropractic because it's natural and it's safe.

Millions of people continue to choose chiropractic because it has worked for them. Ultimately, the choice for healing is yours.

Remember the patient stories you read in chapter 6? Those are real accounts from real people who are now living a healthier, happier, higher-quality of life. They made a choice for healing, and so can you.

A choice for healing is an ongoing process that must be nurtured with a solid commitment and backed up with a clear vision. For some people, progress and improvement with their condition can be slow. Many factors come into play.

Back to health by choice is a journey. Throughout your healing journey, whenever you get discouraged with your progress, do not quit.

Setbacks and upsets are useful reminders that you must choose again to stay on track with your healing journey. If you quit, the journey is over, and you will never cross the finish line. Healing of all forms takes time. It requires a constant cycle of choosing, committing, and choosing again.

Choose → Commit → Choose Again

In closing, my vision for you is for a long-lasting, healthy, happy, and active life. I wish for you an extraordinary life filled with love, happiness, and peace.

To your journey back to health by choice the chiropractic way!

You have the power to heal, which
is but activated by a choice.

—Walter Salubro

Afterword

What Do I Do Next?

Thank you for reading *Back to Health by Choice*. This is an interactive book with free chiropractic patient resources, educational videos, and book updates and upgrades. You will get access to these resources when you visit and register at:

www.BackToHealthByChoice.com/BookBonus

When you visit the website, introduce yourself, leave a comment, and connect with other people like yourself.

In my office, when I share chiropractic success stories with our new patients, they invariably begin to think about their family or friends who are going through similar health problems or pain conditions.

Usually they will say something like this, "Oh, my sister also gets headaches." Or, "My dad has had back pain for years." Or, "That sounds like my friend who has neck pain that shoots into his arm."

Well, if you thought about a friend or family member as you read these stories, then that person should be checked by a chiropractor to see if he or she too can be helped with chiropractic care. And if the person you thought about was you, then you should consider a chiropractic checkup for yourself.

How do you choose a chiropractor? That's a great question. If you received this book as a gift from someone who is currently seeing a chiropractor, ask that person about his or her chiropractor. Referral from a trusted friend or family member is always the best way to choose a chiropractor.

One of the book bonuses on the website is my *"How to Choose a Chiropractor Resource Guide."* It will give you a checklist of what to look for when choosing a chiropractor and what questions to ask when you call a chiropractic office. On the website you will also find chiropractic doctor listings and directories.

Now, if you have friends or family members who are just not ready to get a chiropractic checkup, that's OK. They don't know what you now know after reading this book. Gift them a copy of *Back to Health by Choice* and leave it in their hands, they will make their own choice when they are ready.

B. J. Palmer, the developer of the chiropractic profession, said this:

> We never know how far reaching something we may think, say or do today will affect the lives of millions tomorrow.[1]

Share this book with a loved one who is in pain, suffering, or stressed out and let's see how we can both help affect the life of that person tomorrow.

If you are having challenges finding a chiropractor on your own, then call my office at 905-303-1009. Tell us what city you live in, and my team will personally help you locate a chiropractor from my vast referral network.

If you have any questions about chiropractic care for your particular condition, call me at my office at 905-303-1009 and I will personally extend to you a complimentary fifteen minute telephone consultation.

Do you live in the Greater Toronto Area? My office is located in the City of Vaughan (Maple, Ontario, Canada). You are welcome to come visit us for your chiropractic checkup and begin your journey back to health.

I sincerely hope you found this book enjoyable and enlightening. I wish you a long-lasting, healthy, happy, and active life.

Dr. Walter Salubro

This is an Interactive Book with Free Chiropractic Patient Resources

Please register by visiting the website. Introduce yourself and share your story in the comments. What are your health challenges? What is your *why* for being healthy? What is your *vision* for your life and your health? Are you ready to make a choice for healing? If you are a chiropractic patient, share your chiropractic success story.

You will get free access to these resources:

- A health and stress survey
- The "How to Choose a Chiropractor Resource Guide"
- More chiropractic patient stories
- Educational videos
- Book upgrades and updates
- Tips to conquer stress
- The "Cast Your Vision" Worksheet
- Webinars
- And more...

You will also meet interesting people like yourself.

Visit

www.BackToHealthByChoice.com/BookBonus

Appendix

Frequently Asked Questions about Chiropractic

1. Do I need a referral from my medical doctor to see a chiropractor?

You do not need a referral from your medical doctor to go see a chiropractor. In Canada and the United States, in all provinces and states, chiropractors are primary health-care doctors. The same is true for many other countries around the world. This means you can go visit a chiropractor without a medical referral or prescription.

2. Will the chiropractor "crack me" or "crack my neck"?

Chiropractors do not "crack" anything. The chiropractor delivers a specific, scientific chiropractic adjustment that is aimed at correcting spinal misalignments (also called vertebral subluxations). Sometimes the joints produce a "popping" sound, which is normal during a chiropractic adjustment. The scientific term for that popping sound is "cavitation". Whether or not there is a popping sound, the adjustment is still effective in correcting spinal misalignments.

3. Is a chiropractic adjustment painful?

A chiropractic adjustment is not painful. Chiropractic techniques are applicable to children and infants, which means they are very gentle and safe. Sometimes there could be soreness after an adjustment. This is because the joints, muscles, and tissues are beginning to make changes. When there are changes occurring, you may feel it. It's like going for a run if you haven't run in a very long time—your leg muscles will feel sore. Usually, applying ice to any sore areas for ten minutes will help alleviate the soreness. The soreness tends to get progressively better within the first few visits.

4. Will chiropractic care make my pain worse?

Most people will continue to feel better after they start chiropractic care. In some cases, some people may feel like their symptoms are getting worse. This is usually a sign that the spine and surrounding tissues are beginning to make corrective changes. In a short time, the pain will begin to get progressively better.

5. How long will it take for my condition to get better?

Improvements and progress will vary from patient to patient. With regards to pain, a patient under chiropractic care will begin to experience relief in two to twelve weeks. Keep in mind that this is a general guideline and that results may not be typical. Corrective changes and improvements to global spinal alignment, on the other hand, can take six to twelve months to begin to stabilize and show correction on X-rays. A lot will depend on the degree of spinal misalignment and the extent of existing spinal damage (degenerative arthritis, a.k.a. osteoarthritis). An X-ray analysis will determine the stage of spinal damage, if the spinal misalignment is correctable, and how long it will take to correct. All this information is normally provided by the chiropractor in the report of findings visit.

6. Is chiropractic care only for people who are in pain?

Pain seems to be a primary reason that brings many people to the chiropractic office. However, just because you don't have pain or symptoms doesn't necessarily mean you are healthy. The primary example to illustrate this point is someone who "seems" generally healthy and yet has a massive heart attack. Even though the person felt good and had no pain or symptoms, this person could not have been healthy. He must have had cardiovascular disease even if he was expressing no symptoms or pain. Cardiovascular disease is a sign of poor health. The same is true with the spine and nervous system. Just because you have no pain and are feeling great doesn't mean you don't have vertebral subluxations (spinal misalignments). Many times, vertebral subluxations are unnoticed because there is no pain or expressed symptoms. However, even with no pain, vertebral subluxations will put strain and stress on the nervous system, which is detrimental. The only way to determine if you have vertebral subluxations is to a get a spinal checkup by a chiropractor. If the chiropractor discovers vertebral subluxations, he or she will recommend a care plan to correct them.

Chiropractic care is about correcting vertebral subluxations, removing stress on the nervous system, and restoring the body to optimal function. This means that chiropractic care is also for people who have no pain.

7. Do all chiropractors take X-rays?

An X-ray analysis of the spine is an essential component of the chiropractor's assessment. A spinal X-ray can help determine the state of spinal degeneration, the degree of spinal misalignment, and the prognosis for correction. Also, an X-ray will help dictate adjusting procedures, protocols, and exercise recommendations. Chiropractors will recommend or take X-rays when needed. Some chiropractors who focus on corrective chiropractic care will use X-rays as part of their initial exam and as part of their progress exam to measure changes and improvements.

8. Is it true that once you start going to the chiropractor you have to keep going?

Any patient who starts chiropractic care starts by choice. Any patient who continues to go to a chiropractor does so by choice as well. In life, you don't *have to* do anything you don't want to. Chiropractic is no different. However, many patients who have seen a positive transformation in their life and health continue on with chiropractic care so they can continue to optimize their health. For those people who continue on with chiropractic care, chiropractic becomes an ongoing lifestyle choice, just like going to the gym, brushing your teeth, or eating a nutritious diet. The chiropractor will give the patient his or her best recommendations, and it's up to the patient to follow the recommendations.

9. Is chiropractic covered by insurance plans?

Most health insurance plans cover chiropractic care. Each policy is different. It's best to call your insurance company to determine the exact coverage for chiropractic care under your plan. In most cases, insurance plans do cover chiropractic care.

10. Can I bring my child to the chiropractor?

Yes, you can bring your child to see a chiropractor. Chiropractic care for children is safe, gentle, and effective. Children too can have spinal misalignments. Spinal misalignments in children can occur from falls, like a fall from a changing table, couch, bike, or play structure. However, the most common reason for spinal misalignments in children is trauma at birth. During the birthing process, the baby's neck is often pulled and twisted, causing spinal misalignments and damage to the spinal cord and nerves. When forceps or vacuum extraction instruments are used, the likelihood of spinal misalignments and injury increases. Spinal trauma at birth is a strong reason for children to get a chiropractic checkup. Children respond nicely to chiropractic care, just like adults do.

11. Can I go to the chiropractor if I am pregnant?

Yes, you can receive chiropractic care during any trimester of your pregnancy. Chiropractic care for pregnancy is safe, gentle, and effective in alleviating back pain, hip pain and leg pain due to an increase in weight and a shifting in posture. Chiropractic care for pregnancy helps correct any misalignments and biomechanical imbalances in the pelvic bones. This relieves tension and constraint on the uterus because the ligaments of the uterus are attached to the pelvic bones. This is helpful in creating a safe and ideal environment for the fetus to position itself properly for birth. This can result in a natural, safer, and easier birth for both baby and mom.

A Personal Message from the Author

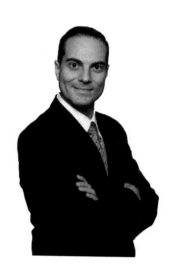

Today, there are many factors that affect people's health and well-being. For instance, stress (from physical, emotional, and chemical sources), poor eating habits, and lack of physical activity are some key factors that contribute to many conditions and health problems. This is posing a huge problem and limiting quality of life in many people. People are getting sicker, not healthier, putting a huge burden in an already overwhelmed health-care system.

This is the reason why our team at Back To Health Chiropractic Centre (located in Maple, Ontario) aims to educate patients and their families to make the best health choices for themselves and their children.

We provide chiropractic care for people who are stressed out, in pain, and are seeking guidance and direction to better health. We have found that preventing illness and disease starts with a healthy spine. So we provide and deliver a systematic approach to chiropractic care that helps alleviate pain, helps relieve stress, and leads you to a healthier, stronger you, now and for the long run.

Our patients get counsel on nutrition and eating habits, exercise recommendations, tips on managing life stresses, guidance for planning life goals, and specific exercises for correcting posture. This well-rounded, vitalistic health-care approach in addition to corrective chiropractic care makes up the foundation of the **5 Pillars of Great Health**—the specific health care model that I teach and promote at Back To Health Chiropractic Centre.

Everyone—adults, children, and infants—deserves the best health care and the best quality of life. Vitality is the natural course for humans. And so, it is our mission to help sick and suffering people of all ages get well with chiropractic care so they can enjoy a long-lasting, healthy, and happy life.

Take the next step toward better health, more happiness, and a higher quality of life. Come visit us and begin your journey back to health.

For your health always,

Dr. Walter Salubro, DC

"Leading you to better health the chiropractic way."
www.iBTHCC.com

Other Seminars, Programs, and Books by Dr. Walter Salubro

5 Pillars of Great Health Seminars:

> **Stress Management Seminar Series**
Self Help Strategies to Conquering Stress

> **Nutrition Mastery Seminar Series**
How to Eat Right for Disease Prevention and Optimal Health

> **Exercise Motivation Seminar Series**
How to Get Lean, Fit and Strong Doing Exercises You Love

> **Vision, Purpose, Goals Seminar Series**
How to Create Your Ideal Life by Design Versus Living Your Life by Default

> **Optimal Spine, Optimal Health Seminar Series**
How to Power Up Your Health the Chiropractic Way

Other Seminars:

- **Back to Health Makeover**
  How to Elevate Your Life with 5 Pillars of Great Health

- **Chiropractic Care for the Wellness Pregnancy**

Home Learning Programs:

- **Stress Management Seminar Series Audio Program**
  (4 CDs and 1 PDF Workbook)

- **Nutrition Mastery Seminar Series Audio Program**
  (4 CDs and 1 PDF Workbook)

Books:

- **3 Step Stretching Plan eBook**
  How to Relieve Stress and Tension in Your Back, Neck and Shoulders

Visit www.WalterSalubro.com for details and registration.

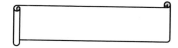

For inquiries, appointments
or further details about seminars...

Call: 905-303-1009

Or Visit:

Back To Health Chiropractic Centre
20 Cranston Park Ave, #6
Maple, Ontario
Tel: 905-303-1009

Visit our clinic website: www.iBTHCC.com

Facebook page for *Back to Health by Choice:*
www.facebook.com/backtohealthbychoice

Visit the book's Facebook page and post your comments and stories.

Speaking Engagements

Dr. Walter Salubro is an engaging and dynamic speaker on topics of chiropractic health and the wellness lifestyle. To have Dr. Salubro appear live at your company, organization, or next event, email speaker@waltersalubro.com or call 905-303-1009.

Notes

Glossary

adjustment: A specific, scientific corrective movement into the joints of the spine for the purpose of correcting vertebral subluxations. An adjustment can be delivered by the chiropractor's hands or with a specialized handheld instrument. The joints of the extremities (arms and legs) can also be adjusted.

corrective chiropractic care: Corrective chiropractic care is an advanced, evidenced-based approach to the correction of spinal misalignments, postural problems, and spinal conditions.

misalignment (spinal misalignment): See *vertebral subluxation.*

nervous system: A body system that is comprised of the central nervous system (brain, brainstem and spinal cord) and the peripheral nervous system. The nervous system controls the function of every other body part, tissue and cell.

parasympathetic nervous system: One of two parts of the autonomic nervous system, it regulates unconscious bodily functions such as pupil constriction, urination, digestion, bowel movements, and saliva production. It stimulates the body's "rest and digest" functions.

sciatic nerve: A large peripheral nerve that emerges from the gluteal area. It is comprised of spinal nerves from the lower back and nerves from the pelvis. The sciatic nerve travels down the back of the thigh. It branches out to reach the structures of the back side of the leg and parts of the foot.

spinal nerves: Peripheral nerves that branch out from both sides of the spinal cord. There are thirty-one pairs of spinal nerves, and they come out from openings on the side of the spine.

spine: A column of twenty-four movable bones, called vertebrae, that extends from the base of the skull to the lower back. It encases and protects the spinal cord.

stressor: An external factor, either real or perceived, that stimulates the body's stress (fight-or-flight) response.

subluxation: See *vertebral subluxation*.

sympathetic nervous system: One of two parts of the autonomic nervous system, it regulates unconscious bodily functions such as heartbeat, pupil dilation, blood-vessel dilation, bronchiole dilation, and sweating. It stimulates the body's 'fight-or-flight' response and helps maintain homeostasis.

vertebra: One of twenty-four bones in the spine.

vertebral subluxation: An abnormal shifting of the spine away from its normal, optimal alignment. It places tension on the nearby spinal nerves and spinal cord, thereby interfering with the normal function of the nervous system.

References

Chapter 3

1. Dorausch, Michael, *"Chiropractic Make Me Prove It"*, PlanetChiropractic.com, http://blog.planetc1.com/chiropractic-make-me-prove-it (Accessed March 10, 2014)

2. Ballard-Barnett, Jessica, *"Sunday Adverts: Benjamin A. Osborne, Chiropractor"*. HistoricIndianapolis.com, http://historicindianapolis.com/sunday-adverts-benjamin-a-osborne-chiropractor (Accessed March 10, 2014)

3. vigor. Oxford Dictionaries. Oxford University Press. http://www.oxforddictionaries.com/definition/american_english/vigor (Accessed January 18, 2015)

Chapter 4

1. Palmer, B. J., *The Bigness of the Fellow Within.* Volume XXII, (1949: repr., Palmer College Of Chiropractic, 1994), p. 572

Chapter 7

1. Mary K., et al, *"Understanding Chronic Stress"*, American Psychological Association, http://www.apa.org/helpcenter/understanding-chronic-stress.aspx (Accessed January 18, 2015).

Chapter 8

1. Statistics Canada. *Canadian Community Health Survey. 2013. Perceived Life Stress, 2013,* http://www.statcan.gc.ca/pub/82-625-x/2014001/article/14023-eng.htm (Accessed January 18, 2015).

2. Anderson, Norman B., et al, *Stress In America: Are Teens Adopting Adults Stress Habits? 2014,* American Psychological Association, http://www.apa.org/news/press/releases/stress/2013/highlights.aspx (Accessed January 18, 2015).

3. Rideout, Victoria M.A., and Ulla G. Foehr, and Donald F. Roberts. *Generation M²: Media In The Lives Of 8-To-18 Year Olds.* A Kaiser Family Foundation Study, January 2010, The Henry J. Kaiser Family Foundation, http://kff.org/other/event/generation-m2-media-in-the-lives-of (Accessed January 18, 2015).

Chapter 9

1. vision. Dictionary.com. *Dictionary.com Unabridged.* Random House, Inc. http://dictionary.reference.com/browse/vision (Accessed January 18, 2015).

2. Allen, James. *As A Man Thinketh,* 1903, The Savoy Publishing Company.

3. Preamble to the Constitution of the World Health Organization as adopted by the International Health Conference, New York, 19-22 June, 1946; signed on 22 July 1946 by the representatives of 61 States (Official Records of the World Health Organization, no. 2, p. 100) and entered into force on 7 April 1948.

http://www.who.int/about/definition/en/print.html (Accessed January 18, 2015).

4. National Center for Health Statistics. *Health, United States, 2013: With Special Feature on Prescription Drugs,* Hyattsville, MD. 2014.

5. Shields, Margot, et al. Statistics Canada. *Fitness of Canadian Adults: Results from the 2007-2009 Canadian Health Measures Survey.* 2010. http://www.statcan.gc.ca/pub/82-003-x/2010001/article/11064-eng.htm (Accessed January 18, 2015)

6. UNICEF Office of Research (2013) "Child Well-being in Rich Countries: A comparative overview", *Innocenti Report Card 11*, UNICEF Office of Research, Florence

Afterword

1. "We never know how far reaching something we may think, say or do today will affect the lives of millions tomorrow." Palmer, B. J. (n.d.). Epigram from the Palmer School of Chiropractic.

Quotations Used In Book

Chapter 4, page 38

Palmer, D. D., *The Chiropractic Adjuster: A Compilation of the Writings of D. D. PALMER by his son B. J. PALMER. D. C.,* Ph. C, The Palmer School of Chiropractic Publishers, Davenport, Iowa, 1921 B. J. Palmer, D. C., Ph. C.

Chapter 6, page 64

Palmer, B. J., *The Bigness of the Fellow Within.* Volume XXII, (1949: repr., Palmer College Of Chiropractic, 1994), p. 572

Index

www.WalterSalubro.com

QUICK ORDER FORM

Fax orders: 905-303-1071. Send this form.

Telephone orders: Call 905-303-1009.
Have your credit card ready.

Email orders: Email orders@waltersalubro.com

Web orders: Visit www.WalterSalubro.com

Postal mail orders: Walter Salubro, 2414 Major Mackenzie Dr, PO Box 96533 Maple, Ontario, L6A 1W5, Canada

Bulk orders: Visit www.WalterSalubro.com for bulk pricing.

Please send the following books or home learning programs. I understand that I may return any of them for a full refund, for any reason.

_____

_____

Name: _____

Address: _____

City: _____ Province/State: _____

Postal code/Zip: _____Telephone: _____

Email address: _____

Sales tax: Canadian residents please add your applicable GST/HST to all products and shipping/handling.

Shipping & Handling:

Canada: $5.95 per book/product.

U.S.: $11.95 per book/product.

For multiple products, call for S&H.

International: Call for S&H pricing.

Payment: ☐Check ☐Visa ☐MasterCard ☐AMEX ☐Discover

Name on card: _____

Card #: _____

Expiry date: _____ CVC code: _____

www.WalterSalubro.com

QUICK ORDER FORM

Fax orders: 905-303-1071. Send this form.

Telephone orders: Call 905-303-1009.
Have your credit card ready.

Email orders: Email orders@waltersalubro.com

Web orders: Visit www.WalterSalubro.com

Postal mail orders: Walter Salubro, 2414 Major Mackenzie Dr, PO Box 96533 Maple, Ontario, L6A 1W5, Canada

Bulk orders: Visit www.WalterSalubro.com for bulk pricing.

Please send the following books or home learning programs. I understand that I may return any of them for a full refund, for any reason.

_____

_____

Name: _____

Address: _____

City: _____ Province/State: _____

Postal code/Zip: _____Telephone: _____

Email address: _____

Sales tax: Canadian residents please add your applicable GST/HST to all products and shipping/handling.

Shipping & Handling:

Canada: $5.95 per book/product.

U.S.: $11.95 per book/product.

For multiple products, call for S&H.

International: Call for S&H pricing.

Payment: ☐Check ☐Visa ☐MasterCard ☐AMEX ☐Discover

Name on card: _____

Card #: _____

Expiry date: _____ CVC code: _____

www.WalterSalubro.com

QUICK ORDER FORM

Fax orders: 905-303-1071. Send this form.

Telephone orders: Call 905-303-1009.
Have your credit card ready.
Email orders: Email orders@waltersalubro.com
Web orders: Visit www.WalterSalubro.com
Postal mail orders: Walter Salubro, 2414 Major Mackenzie Dr, PO Box 96533 Maple, Ontario, L6A 1W5, Canada
Bulk orders: Visit www.WalterSalubro.com for bulk pricing.

Please send the following books or home learning programs. I understand that I may return any of them for a full refund, for any reason.

_____

_____

Name: _____

Address: _____

City: _____ Province/State: _____

Postal code/Zip: _____Telephone: _____

Email address: _____

Sales tax: Canadian residents please add your applicable GST/HST to all products and shipping/handling.

Shipping & Handling:

Canada: $5.95 per book/product.

U.S.: $11.95 per book/product.

For multiple products, call for S&H.

International: Call for S&H pricing.

Payment: ☐Check ☐Visa ☐MasterCard ☐AMEX ☐Discover

Name on card: _____

Card #: _____

Expiry date: _____ CVC code: _____